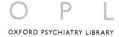

OXFORD PSYCHIATRY LIBRARY

Psychedelics as Psychiatric Medications

T0355327

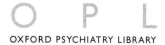

OXFORD PSYCHIATRY LIBRARY

Psychedelics as Psychiatric Medications

Edited by

David Nutt

Edmond J. Safra Prof of Neuropsychopharmacology and
director of the Centre for Psychedelic Research, Department of
Psychiatry, Division of Brain Sciences, Commonwealth Building,
Hammersmith Hospital, UK

David Castle

Scientific Director, Centre for Complex Interventions, Centre
for Addiction and Mental Health; and Professor, Department of
Psychiatry, The University of Toronto, Canada

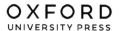

OXFORD
UNIVERSITY PRESS

OXFORD
UNIVERSITY PRESS

Great Clarendon Street, Oxford, OX2 6DP,
United Kingdom

Oxford University Press is a department of the University of Oxford.
It furthers the University's objective of excellence in research, scholarship,
and education by publishing worldwide. Oxford is a registered trade mark of
Oxford University Press in the UK and in certain other countries

First Edition published in 2023

Published in the United States of America by Oxford University Press
198 Madison Avenue, New York, NY 10016, United States of America

British Library Cataloguing in Publication Data

Data available

Library of Congress Control Number: 2022952041

ISBN 978–0–19–286360–7

DOI: 10.1093/med/9780192863607.001.0001

Printed and bound by
CPI Group (UK) Ltd, Croydon, CR0 4YY

Preface

We are very pleased to present this book, which provides a current appraisal of a very fast-moving field. We are gratified by having chapters by thought leaders from across the world, who have given a good sense of where we came from, where we are, and where we are going, in terms of psychedelics as treatments for psychiatric maladies and addictions. It should be noted that this book has embraced a very broad definition of 'psychedelics and related agents', including ketamine (a dissociative anaesthetic) and N-methyl-3,4-methylenedioxyamphetamine (MDMA, an entactogen), along with the 'classic' psychedelics (e.g. psilocybin, D-lysergic acid diethylamide (LSD), dimethyltryptamine (DMT), ibogaine, and mescaline), as well as some 'lesser-known' agents (muscimol, salvinorin A, mescaline, 2C-B, and 5-methoxy-DMT). This has been in part a response to the fact that these agents are all novel in terms of mechanisms of action; that all entail a rethinking of traditional therapeutic 'wrap around', in terms of the psychotherapeutic component (which, for ease, we refer to as 'psychedelic-assisted psychotherapy' or PAP), and that all are in a stage of excited discovery. Indeed, the excitement associated with the revisiting of these agents as potential treatments for mental health and addictions is evidenced by a massive surge in publications, lectures, and media coverage.

We believe this book will be helpful to specialists and nonspecialists alike. The science and art of psychedelic psychiatry are presented, along with due cautions and concerns for how the future of this fascinating group of compounds can, along with psychotherapeutic support, help patients with a range of mental health and addiction problems.

David Nutt and David Castle
February 2022

Contents

List of abbreviations *viii*

1 Historical overview   1
  Chase Thompson and Ishrat M. Husain

2 The psychotherapeutic component of psychedelic medicine   **15**
  Laurie Higbed and Ben Sessa

3 Psilocybin   **25**
  James J. Rucker and David Erritzoe

4 MDMA   **39**
  Michael C. Mithoefer and David E. Presti

5 Lysergic acid diethylamide: In search of the wonder drug   **53**
  Mihai Avram, Felix Müller, and Stefan Borgwardt

6 Ayahuasca   **65**
  Daniel Perkins, Simon G. D. Ruffell, and Jerome Sarris

7 Ibogaine: Ibogaine therapy as a method of care treatment for
  opioid dependence   **75**
  Deborah C. Mash

8 Other psychedelics   **95**
  James Linden and Daniel Robin

9 Ketamine   **103**
  Joshua D. Di Vincenzo, Joshua D. Rosenblat, and Roger S. McIntyre

10 Risks and adverse events associated with the use of psychedelics **113**
   Joanna C. Neill, Mohammed Shahid, Rosalind Gittins, Anne K. Schlag,
   and Frank I. Tarazi

11 Psychedelics as psychiatric medicines: Current challenges and
   future prospects   **131**
   David Castle, Nicole Ledwos, and David Nutt

Index *147*

List of abbreviations

5-HT	Serotonin
ACE	Adverse childhood experience
ACLS	Advanced Cardiac Life Support
AR	Augmented reality
ASI	Addiction Severity Index
BD	Bipolar disorder
BDNF	Brain-derived neurotrophic factor
BOLD	Blood oxygen level-dependent
CADSS	Clinician-Administered Dissociative States Scale
CAPS	Clinician-Administered PTSD Scale
CBCT	Cognitive-behavioural conjoint therapy
CDLIN	Controlled Drug Local Intelligence Networks
CEQ	Challenging Experiences Questionnaire
CNS	Central nervous system
CRP	C-reactive protein
CSA	Controlled Substances Act
DAAC	Drug Abuse Advisory Committee
DMN	Default-mode network
DMT	N, N-dimethyltrpyamine
DOS	Delirium observation scale
DSM-5	*Diagnostic and Statistical Manual of Mental Disorders*, fifth ed.
EBI	Emotional Breakthrough Inventory
EC	Endothelial cell
ECG	Electrocardiogram
EEG	Electroencephalogram
EMA	European Medicines Agency
FDA	Food and Drug Administration
FM	Frequency Modulation
GABA	γ-Aminobutyric acid
GERD	Gastroesophageal reflux
GLP	Good Laboratory Practice
GPCR	G-protein coupled receptor
HNK	Human Natural Killer
IASC	Inventory of Altered Self-Capacities
IBN	Intrinsic brain networks

ICD-10	International Classification of Diseases, tenth ed.
IPT	interpersonal psychotherapy
LSD	D-lysergic acid diethylamide
MAOI	Monoamine oxidase-A enzyme inhibitor
MAPS	Multidisciplinary Association for Psychedelic Studies
MDA	3,4-Methylenedioxyamphetamine
MDD	Major depressive disorder
MDMA	3,4-Methyl-enedioxy-methamphetamine
MEG	Magnetoencephalography
MEQ	Mystical Experiences Questionnaire
MHRA	Medicines and Healthcare products Regulatory Agency
MI	Motivational interviewing
NHMRC	National Health and Medical research Council
NICE	National Institute for Health and Care Excellence
NIDA	National Institute on Drug Abuse
NIMH	National Institutes for Mental Health
NMDA	N-methyl-D-aspartate
NMDAR	N-methyl D-aspartate receptor
NREM	Non-Rapid Eye Movement
OWS	Opioid Withdrawal Syndrome
PAP	Psychedelic-assisted psychotherapy
PCP	Phencyclidine
PET	Positron emission tomography
PFC	Prefrontal cortex
PIHKAL	Phenethylamines I Have Known And Loved
PIS	Psychological Insight Scale
PK	Pharmacokinetics
PKC	Protein kinase C
PTSD	Posttraumatic stress disorder
RAM	Reward Activation Model
RBANS	Repeatable Battery for the Assessment of Neuropsychological Status
RCT	Randomized controlled trial
REMS	Risk Evaluation and Mitigation Strategy
SA	Substance Abuse
SAE	Serious adverse event
SCS	Self-Compassion Scale
SERT	Serotonin transporter
SNRI	Serotonin and noradrenaline reuptake inhibitor

SOWS	Subjective Opioid Withdrawal Scale
SRI	Serotonin Reuptake Inhibitor
SSRI	Selective serotonin reuptake inhibitor
TCA	Tricyclic antidepressants
TD	Tardive Dyskinesia
TdP	Torsade des Points
TEAE	Treatment-emergent adverse event
TRD	Treatment-resistant depression
VA	Veterans Affairs
VSMC	Vascular smooth muscle cell

CHAPTER 1

Historical overview

Chase Thompson and Ishrat M. Husain

KEY POINTS

* Psychedelic compounds have been used among different cultural groups for millenia.
* Between the 1950s and 1970, psychedelics showed promise in early clinical trials for the treatment of various psychiatric disorders.
* The classification of psychedelic compounds as Schedule 1 drugs and the resultant decline in scientific research were primarily driven by political motivations as opposed to evidence of harm.
* Psychedelic science is experiencing a resurgence because of encouraging findings from small contemporary studies that suggest efficacy for the treatment of psychiatric disorders.

Terminology

The 'classic' psychedelics are a group of compounds that share similar pharmacologic and psychotropic characteristics. They include psilocybin, D-lysergic acid diethylamide (LSD), dimethyltryptamine (DMT), ibogaine, and mescaline. Notable exclusions from this group are MDMA and ketamine, which have overlapping but sufficiently distinct pharmacologic profiles (Roseman et al., 2014; Nichols, 2016; Nutt, 2019) but which we do include in this book, for reasons articulated in Chapter 11. The term 'psychedelic' is derived from ancient Greek and translates roughly to '*mind-manifesting*' (Savage, 1964)—it was first proposed by a psychiatrist named Humphry Osmond in 1956 (Osmond, 1957). Other terms have been proposed, including 'hallucinogen', or 'psychotomimetic', though these terms are arguably too simplistic or inaccurate, or imply that the psychedelics are wholly pathogenic (Nichols, 2016). The descriptor 'psychedelic' seems to come closest to describing the complex psychological phenomena evoked by these compounds. Notably, the fifth and most recent iteration of the *Diagnostic and Statistical Manual of Mental Disorders* (DSM-5), and the *International Classification of Diseases* (or ICD-10) continue to use the term 'hallucinogen', as do some scientists and clinicians.

'The first wave': the origins and ancient use of psychedelic compounds

Psychedelic compounds are ubiquitous within the natural world. DMT, for one, has been identified and isolated from a vast array of different plant and animal species (Winstock et al., 2014; Halpern, 2004; Shulgin and Shulgin, 1997; Cameron & Olson, 2018), and has even been identified within the mammalian brain (Christian et al., 1977; Barker et al., 2012; Dean et al., 2019). Similarly, psilocybin-producing fungi have been found around the globe, and across multiple fungal lineages (Andersson et al., 2009; Reynolds et al., 2018). Despite their ubiquity, the function that these compounds serve in nature is only partially understood. Psilocybin, for example, is an alkaloid that can be found throughout the mushroom body and is known to comprise up to 2% of the dry weight of the mushroom (Beug & Bigwood, 1982). The prevalence of psilocybin among mushroom species (and within an individual mushroom) suggests that psilocybin has an important functional role. Akin to other naturally occurring alkaloids (e.g. caffeine, atropine), psilocybin may, in part, serve a protective role for the fungi by reducing the appetite of insects who attempt to consume them (Awan et al., 2018; Reynolds et al., 2018; Wink, 2020). Humans experience similar reductions in appetite after ingesting psychedelic compounds (Holze et al., 2022; Studerus et al., 2011), though it is unclear whether the associated psychological experience is simply an accidental by-product of the appetite-suppressing effects or whether the psychedelic effects are functionally independent and important.

Terence McKenna, a popular mystic and ethnobotanist, believed that the psychedelic effects of psilocybin-containing fungi were a vital component of human evolution. He coined the 'Stoned Ape' theory to describe how the consumption of psilocybin-producing mushrooms may have altered the evolutionary course of the human brain and cognition. His theory is based on the last 100,000 years (or more), when cattle had become a dietary staple for early nomadic humans. Consequently, these early humans would have tracked herds of cattle, encountered, and consumed psilocybin-containing mushrooms growing in the cattle's dung (McKenna, 1999). McKenna proposed that regular consumption of these fungi, along with the associated psychedelic experience, was a major driving force behind the rapid cognitive and frontal cortical expansion of *Homo erectus*—a development which paved the way to modern-day *Homo sapiens*. Specifically, he believed that psilocybin facilitated the development of speech, enhanced creativity, hunting, and reproduction within psilocybin-consuming groups (among other benefits). As a result, groups of early humans who consumed psilocybin-containing mushrooms held an evolutionary advantage over those who did not, and such advantages would have led to greater flourishing and expansion of these groups. His theory has largely been ignored by the scientific community because there is limited evidence to support or refute its tenets. Nonetheless the 'Stoned Ape' theory remains an interesting conjecture, suggesting that the ingestion of psychedelic compounds was a fundamental and widespread practice among early humans, one from which modern-day humans have largely deviated.

One argument that indirectly supports McKenna's theory is the widespread use of psychedelic compounds among ancient and indigenous cultures, often as a component of spiritual or medicinal practices (Walter & Fridman, 2004; MAPS, 2007; Doblin et al., 2019; George et al., 2021). In a region crossing Mexico and Texas, archaeological and carbon-dating evidence suggest that the indigenous people in this area were consuming mescaline-containing cacti around 10,500 BP (Adovasio & Fry, 1976). Across the world, in a cave in Algeria, there is a cave painting that depicts a psilocybin-containing mushroom that is estimated to be around 7000–9000 BP (Samorini, 1992). Similarly, cave paintings of psychedelic fungi have been found in Spain as well (Akers et al., 2011). In ancient Greece, it has been hypothesized that the *Eleusinian mysteries*, a legendary set of secret religious ceremonies where participants often experienced deep revelations and hallucinations, were inspired by psychedelic compounds present in the wine (Wasson, 2008). Together, these pieces of evidence suggest that psychedelics played an important role within ancient and indigenous cultures, and there are likely many more instances than we have available evidence for. The use of psychedelics by indigenous peoples and ancient civilizations has been coined the 'the first wave' (Austin et al., 2017).

The discovery of LSD and initial wave of psychedelic research

The original synthesis of LSD in 1938 by Albert Hofmann, a Swiss chemist, was a crucial event in psychedelic history (Hofmann & Ott, 1980). He synthesized LSD from ergotamine, an alkaloid-derivative of ergot, which is a fungus that grows on rye grains (Liester, 2014). At the time, Hofmann was in search of a medication that could be used as a cardio-respiratory stimulant—he was not aware of the potent psychoactive effects of LSD until he mistakenly ingested the substance through his fingertips five years later. The discovery was one of a few seminal events that led to the reintroduction of psychedelics to Western society. Another was when Gordon Wasson, an American banker, travelled to Oaxaca, Mexico, and met with Maria Sabina, a Mazatec *curandera* (medicine woman). She shared with him a sacred Mesoamerican ritual called *velada*, which involved the ingestion of psilocybin (Wasson, 1961). As a result of his experience, Wasson wrote the popular article 'Seeking the Magic Mushroom' in *Life* magazine in 1957, which further added to the growing enthusiasm for psychedelics in Western society (Wasson, 1957).

Soon after the discovery of LSD, the field of psychiatry—which at the time was primarily focused on psychotherapy and psychoanalysis—became fascinated by the compound and its therapeutic potential (Belouin & Henningfield, 2018). LSD and psilocybin were brought to market by Sandoz pharmaceuticals under the trade names Delysid, and Indocybin, respectively, and an era of clinical study commenced. Researchers quickly noticed that LSD produced an interesting array of psychological effects, including euphoria, anxiety, dissociation, increased empathy, visual perceptual changes, and others (Savage, 1952; Deshon et al., 1952; Freedman, 1968). Some early studies of LSD included individuals with schizophrenia, where reports indicate that the study participants exhibited worsening of symptoms, such as intensification of delusions and preoccupations, increased vividness of pre-existing hallucinations (Cholden et al., 1955), or a 'regression to a prime stage' of their psychosis (Anastasopoulos & Photiades, 1962). On the other hand, individuals with prominent negative symptoms of schizophrenia seemed to be relatively immune to the effects of LSD (Cholden et al., 1955).

Although many of these studies were methodologically limited and unethical by today's standards, it was increasingly believed that LSD (and psychedelics more broadly) had limited therapeutic benefit, and evident potential harms for individuals with schizophrenia or bipolar disorder (Denber & Merlis, 1955; Fink et al., 1966; Frosch et al., 1965; Rucker et al., 2018). The observation that LSD seemed to reproduce or provoke certain aspects of the psychotic experience was reason enough for some to classify LSD as a 'psychotomimetic', and provided support for the idea that aspects of psychotic illness were biologically based (Geyer & Vollenweider, 2008). Interestingly, the observation that the psychological effects induced by LSD were related to activation of brain-based serotonin receptors, led to greater interest in the neurotransmitter and ignited the field of serotonin neuroscience in the 1950s (Nichols, 2016).

While studies were ongoing in schizophrenia, psychedelics were also being investigated for potential therapeutic effects in addictions and internalizing disorders such as depression, anxiety, and obsessive-compulsive disorder (Sandison et al., 1954; Rucker et al., 2018; Nichols, 2020). In these disorders, psychedelics seemed to have greater therapeutic success and less potential harms (Rucker et al., 2016). For example, studies of psychedelics in individuals with disordered alcohol use showed promise in helping individuals slow down, or even stop, dangerous patterns of drinking (Jensen, 1962). However, similar to the trials of psychedelics in schizophrenia, many of these studies were poorly designed, making their overall conclusions uncertain (Rucker et al., 2018). During these initial studies an important observation emerged—that the environment encompassing one's psychedelic experience seemed to be an important factor in the clinical outcome. For example, the availability of a support person, involvement of music during the session, or the use of psychotherapy, were all observed to influence the psychedelic experience and were associated with the degree of therapeutic effectiveness (Cholden et al., 1955; Robbins et al., 1967; Carhart-Harris et al., 2018).

The end of the first wave of psychedelic research

During the initial wave of psychedelic research, there were roughly more than a hundred studies carried out with Delysid (or LSD) (Nutt & Carhart-Harris,

Box 1.1 Factors leading to the end of the second wave

- Sandoz patents on Indocybin and Delysid ended
- Psychedelics became associated with the anti–Vietnam War movement and became a target of government scrutiny and regulation to criminalize political dissidents as 'drug users'
- Media coverage of psychedelic compounds focused on adverse outcomes and unethical use by the CIA as part of 'MKUltra'
- Psychedelics became classified as Schedule I drugs under the UN convention, which defined them as having no accepted medical use, making ethics approval and research funding difficult to obtain

2021) and an additional hundred studies with Indocybin (or synthetic psilocybin) (Nichols, 2020). However, as quickly as this initial wave of studies emerged, things came to an abrupt halt in the early 1970s as a result of several coinciding factors (see Box 1.1). For one, the patents on Delysid and Indocybin expired in the 1960s, and therefore, Sandoz' financial incentive to fund further clinical trials diminished—though a significant proportion of funding for psychedelic trials also came from the National Institutes for Mental Health in the United States (NIMH) (Bonson, 2018).

Perhaps a more powerful influence associated with the decline in psychedelic research was the shifting public and political narratives around these compounds. Psychedelics had 'leaked out of the laboratory' in the United States and became part of the hippie subculture and anti–Vietnam War movement (Sessa, 2012; Nichols, 2016). At the time, the anti-war movement was placing increasing pressures on the Nixon administration to end the unpopular war. In response, the Nixon administration sought to discredit the anti-war movement by labelling dissidents as drug users and criminals (Schultz, 2013; Baker, 2017). The Nixon administration passed the Controlled Substances Act (CSA), a federal drug policy that allowed the government to closely regulate the use and distribution of psychedelic compounds (Nutt et al., 2013; Belouin & Henningfield, 2018). Many presumed that the government had ulterior political motives in their implementation of the CSA and subsequent 'war on drugs' that followed, yet it was not until the interview of one of Richard Nixon's top presidential aids, John Ehrlichman, that this sentiment was confirmed (Baum, 2016; LoBianco, 2016):

"We knew we couldn't make it illegal to be either against the war or black, but by getting the public to associate the hippies with marijuana and blacks with heroin. And then criminalizing both heavily, we could disrupt those communities ... We could arrest their leaders, raid their homes, break up their meetings, and vilify them night after night on the evening news. Did we know we were lying about the drugs? Of course we did."

—John Ehrlichman 1994

In addition to the increasing government regulation and criminalization of psyche-delic compounds, fears grew regarding their associated physiologic and psycho-logical harms. Reports in the media claimed, often without sufficient evidence, that LSD could lead to death by suicide, cause chromosomal damage (New York Times, 1971) or cause deformed offspring (New York Times, 1967). Concerns were also raised about the possibility of 'flashbacks' after use of LSD, that is, re-experiencing visual perceptual changes long after the effects of the substance had worn off. Although the legitimacy of flashbacks is still a topic of debate, the phe-nomenon was added to the DSM-III-R as 'post-hallucinogen perception disorder' in 1986, and would later become renamed 'hallucinogen persisting perception disorder' in the DSM-5 (Halpern & Pope, 2003; Orsolini et al., 2017).

Psychedelics continued to be dragged down a morally dubious path when Timothy Leary, a psychologist and psychedelic advocate working at Harvard University, was fired by the university in 1963 for allegedly providing psychedelics to his students. Leary's fervent promotion for the use of psychedelics, and his os-tensible libertinism, led him to be labelled the 'most dangerous man in America' by former President Nixon (Minutaglio & Davis, 2018)—although others have challenged this supposed labelling (Gunther, 2020). Possibly one of the most disturbing revelations related to psychedelics was their use by the CIA in illegal mind-control and torture-based experiments as a part of project 'MKUltra' (US Senate, 1977; Szalavitz, 2012).

While psychedelics became strictly regulated under the CSA, the public was persuaded that these strict regulations were both rational and necessary. Within the United States, psychedelics were classified as 'Schedule I' substances, meaning that they were considered to have no legitimate medical use and a high potential for abuse and harm (Bonson, 2018). Many countries around the globe followed suit with similar drug policies, in large part due to pressures from the United Nations (Khan, 1979; Rucker, 2015; Walsh, 2016). Although it could be reason-ably argued that *some* degree of regulatory control was warranted due to reports of adverse outcomes associated with psychedelic use, their classification under Schedule I status halted any further research that could have provided a more complete understanding of their potential harms and benefits (Smart & Bateman, 1967; Nutt et al., 2013; Nichols & Grob, 2018). Under Schedule I status, funding for psychedelic research was essentially unobtainable, and the field came to a standstill that would go on for several decades (Rucker et al., 2018).

The modern psychedelic renaissance or the 'third wave'

In the 1990s, a group of scientists reignited the field of psychedelic research after a near twenty-five-year pause (Carhart-Harris & Goodwin, 2017; Rucker et al., 2018). These groups were led by Leo Hermle in Germany (Hermle et al., 1992; Hermle et al., 1998), Rick Strassman in the United States (Strassman & Qualls, 1994), and Franz Vollenweider in Switzerland (Vollenweider et al., 1997; Vollenweider et al., 1998). To get their research approved in a time of strict

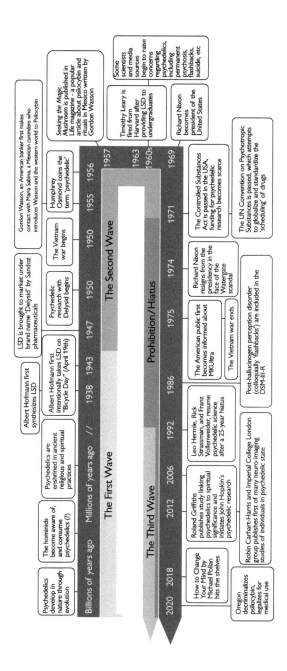

Figure 1.1 A timeline of psychedelic use throughout history, separated into the first, second, and third waves; the third wave has continued despite ongoing restrictions from the prohibition era.

regulation, these scientists had to work closely with governmental regulatory authorities and advocate for the value of their work (Strassman, 2018). Still, after twenty-five years of hiatus, the psychedelics had remained compounds of interest in the field of mental health, in part, due to the dearth of other new and effective psychiatric treatments (Nutt, 2020).

The 'third wave', while still ongoing, has had some important differences from the second. For one, more attention has been paid to research methodology, such that the outcomes from more recent studies have generally been more reliable and well-defined (Rucker et al., 2018). In addition, and as detailed in other chapters in this book, modern technologies, not available during the second wave, such as functional magnetic resonance (or fMRI), have enabled researchers to gain fascinating insights into the ways in which these compounds affect brain function (Carhart-Harris et al., 2012; Carhart-Harris et al., 2014; Carhart-Harris & Friston, 2019). Lastly, many third-wave studies have been relatively small and primarily focused on safety and tolerability of psychedelic-assisted psychotherapy, rather than efficacy per se (Schunemann et al., 2006; Nutt, 2021). Along these lines, most recent studies have had exclusion criteria for psychotic and bipolar-based illnesses. Given the historical pitfalls of psychedelic research, third-wave researchers have been intensely aware of the potential setbacks that could occur from work lacking sufficient scientific rigour or attention to safety.

In the small contemporary trials completed thus far, it appears that psychedelic-assisted psychotherapy is safe and potentially effective in the treatment of various mental and substance use disorders (Johnson, 2019; Andersen et al., 2021). As an overview, studies have suggested therapeutic efficacy of psychedelic-assisted psychotherapy in treating depressive disorders (Carhart-Harris et al., 2016; Carhart-Harris et al., 2021), anxiety and depression associated with advanced or life-threatening cancers (Ross et al., 2016; Griffiths et al., 2016); smoking cessation (Johnson et al., 2017), reducing alcohol use (Bogenschutz et al., 2015); and evoking mystical experiences (Griffiths et al., 2006; Griffiths et al., 2011; Griffiths et al., 2018). However, larger studies with rigorous clinical trial design and greater statistical power are needed to more accurately determine the safety and efficacy of psychedelic-assisted psychotherapy (see Chapter 11).

Promising early data for psychedelic-assisted psychotherapy and evidence for physiologic safety (Johansen & Krebs, 2015; Nichols & Grob, 2016) have led to pressures for reduced government regulation, and increased access for researchers, prescribers, and the general public (Johnson et al., 2008; Rucker, 2015). The degree to which psychedelics should be deregulated remains a topic of disagreement among experts (Strassman, 2018; Johnson et al., 2018), and yet while government and scientific communities struggle to find an optimum of regulation, the public has not been patiently waiting. Online and media portrayals of psychedelics, where they have been described as mood, cognitive, or productivity enhancers, have led to increasing popularity and an uptick in use, particularly of 'micro-dosing' regimens (Dean, 2017; Hogan, 2017; Lea et al., 2020; Yockey et al., 2020). In addition, private businesses have forged ahead in making psychedelic compounds widely accessible through illegal online stores and dispensaries in what has become a booming and unregulated market (Aday et al., 2019; The Economist, 2019). Nonetheless, psychedelic use remains relatively rare, where one-year prevalence in the United States was less than 1% in 2018 (Yockey et al., 2020), though this figure may well go up due to increasing ease of access in obtaining psychedelic compounds, the degree of public interest in psychedelic research, and a cultural zeitgeist that is fascinated with self-improvement and self-actualization.

Overall, psychedelics have played an intriguing and complex role in the history of humankind. Their powerful psychological effects have fascinated some, and evoked fear and disgust in others, to the extent that these compounds have become and remain criminalized throughout the world. Yet, the growing appreciation of the need for new treatments in mental health, coupled with changing attitudes towards psychedelic drugs, has set the scene for a new frontier in psychedelic research. The time is opportune to conduct further well-designed, scientifically rigorous, mechanistic clinical trials of these compounds to inform clinical translation. Only time and further study will reveal the role these compounds have to play in psychiatric care and society at large. The rest of this book takes up this story, addressing individual compounds, looking at the current state of the science, and scoping future directions, opportunities, and potential pitfalls.

REFERENCES

Aday JS, Bloesch EK, Davoli CC (2019) A year of expansion in psychedelic research, industry, and deregulation. Drug Science, Policy and Law 6:2050324520974484.

Adovasio JM, Fry GF (1976) Prehistoric psychotropic drug use in northeastern Mexico and Trans-Pecos Texas. Economic Botany 30:94–96.

Akers BP, Ruiz JF, Piper A, Ruck CA (2011) A prehistoric mural in Spain depicting neurotropic psilocybe mushrooms? Economic Botany 65:121–128.

Anastasopoulos G, Photiades H (1962) Effects of LSD-25 on relatives of schizophrenic patients. Journal of Mental Science 108:95–98.

Andersen KA, Carhart-Harris R, Nutt DJ, Erritzoe D (2021) Therapeutic effects of classic serotonergic psychedelics: a systematic review of modern-era clinical studies. Acta Psychiatrica Scandinavica 143:101–118.

Andersson C, Kristinsson J, Gry J (2009) Occurrence and use of hallucinogenic mushrooms containing psilocybin alkaloids. Nordic Council of Ministers.

Austin P, Tudorie V, Stone R, et al. (2017) What is the Third Wave of Psychedelics? Available at: https://thethirdwave.co/about/ (accessed November 5, 2021).

Awan AR, Winter JM, Turner D, et al. (2018) Convergent evolution of psilocybin biosynthesis by psychedelic mushrooms. BioRxiv 374199.

Baker P (2017) Nixon tried to spoil Johnson's Vietnam peace talks in '68, notes show. New York Times.

Barker SA, McIlhenny EH, Strassman R (2012) A critical review of reports of endogenous psychedelic N, N-dimethyltryptamines in humans: 1955–2010. Drug Testing and Analysis 4:617–635.

Baum D (2016) Legalize it all. Harper's Magazine 24:21–32.

Belouin SJ, Henningfield JE (2018) Psychedelics: where we are now, why we got here, what we must do. Neuropharmacology 142:7–19.

Beug MW, Bigwood J (1982) Psilocybin and psilocin levels in twenty species from seven genera of wild mushrooms in the Pacific Northwest, USA. Journal of Ethnopharmacology 5:271–285.

Bogenschutz MP, Forcehimes AA, Pommy JA, et al. (2015) Psilocybin-assisted treatment for alcohol dependence: a proof-of-concept study. Journal of Psychopharmacology 29:289–299.

Bonson KR (2018) Regulation of human research with LSD in the United States (1949–1987). Psychopharmacology 2018:591–604.

Cameron LP, Olson DE (2018) Dark classics in chemical neuroscience: N, N-Dimethyltryptamine (DMT). ACS Chemical Neuroscience 9:2344–2357.

Carhart-Harris RL, Erritzoe D, Williams T, et al. (2012) Neural correlates of the psychedelic state as determined by fMRI studies with psilocybin. Proceedings of the National Academy of Sciences 109:2138–2143.

Carhart-Harris RL, Leech R, Hellyer PJ, et al. (2014) The entropic brain: a theory of conscious states informed by neuroimaging research with psychedelic drugs. Frontiers in Human Neuroscience 8:20.

Carhart-Harris RL, Bolstridge M, Rucker J, et al. (2016) Psilocybin with psychological support for treatment-resistant depression: an open-label feasibility study. Lancet Psychiatry 3:619–627.

Carhart-Harris RL, Goodwin GM (2017) The therapeutic potential of psychedelic drugs: past, present, and future. Neuropsychopharmacology 42:2105–2113.

Carhart-Harris RL, Roseman L, Haijen E, et al. (2018) Psychedelics and the essential importance of context. Journal of Psychopharmacology 32:725–731.

Carhart-Harris RL, Friston, KJ (2019) REBUS and the anarchic brain: toward a unified model of the brain action of psychedelics. Pharmacological Reviews 71:316–344.

Carhart-Harris R, Giribaldi B, Watts R, et al. (2021) Trial of psilocybin versus escitalopram for depression. New England Journal of Medicine 384:1402–1411.

Cholden LS, Kurland A, Savage C (1955) Clinical reactions and tolerance to LSD in chronic schizophrenia. Journal of Nervous and Mental Disease 122:211–221.

Christian ST, Harrison R, Quayle E, et al. (1977) The in vitro identification of dimethyltryptamine (DMT) in mammalian brain and its characterization as a possible endogenous neuroregulatory agent. Biochemical Medicine 18:164–183.

Dean J (2017) Micro-dosing: the drug habit your boss is gonna love. GQ Magazine.

Dean JG, Liu T, Huff S, et al. (2019) Biosynthesis and extracellular concentrations of N, N-dimethyltryptamine (DMT) in mammalian brain. Scientific Reports 9:1–11.

Denber HC, Merlis S (1955) Studies on mescaline I: action in schizophrenic patients. Psychiatric Quarterly 29:421–429.

Deshon HJ, Rinkel M, Solomon HC (1952) Mental changes experimentally produced by LSD (d-lysergic acid diethylamide tartrate). Psychiatric Quarterly 26:33–53.

Doblin RE, Christiansen M, Jerome L, Burge B (2019) The past and future of psychedelic science: an introduction to this issue. Journal of Psychoactive Drugs 51:93–97.

Fink M, Simeon J, Haque W, Itil T (1966) Prolonged adverse reactions to LSD in psychotic subjects. Archives of General Psychiatry 15:450–454.

Freedman DX (1968) On the use and abuse of LSD. Archives of General Psychiatry 18:330–347.

Frosch WA, Robbins ES, Stern M (1965) Untoward reactions to lysergic acid diethylamide (LSD) resulting in hospitalization. New England Journal of Medicine 273:1235–1239.

Gael S (2021) Expert Q&A: MAPS and psychedelic-assisted psychotherapy. Depression.

George DR, Hanson R, Wilkinson D, Garcia-Romeu A (2021) Ancient roots of today's emerging renaissance in psychedelic medicine. Culture, Medicine, and Psychiatry 1–14.

Geyer MA, Vollenweider FX (2008) Serotonin research: contributions to understanding psychoses. Trends in Pharmacological Sciences 29:445–453.

Griffiths RR, Richards WA, McCann U, Jesse R (2006) Psilocybin can occasion mystical-type experiences having substantial and sustained personal meaning and spiritual significance. Psychopharmacology 187:268–283.

Griffiths RR, Johnson MW, Richards WA, et al. (2011) Psilocybin occasioned mystical-type experiences: immediate and persisting dose-related effects. Psychopharmacology 218:649–665.

Griffiths RR, Johnson MW, Carducci MA (2016) Psilocybin produces substantial and sustained decreases in depression and anxiety in patients with life-threatening cancer: a randomized double-blind trial. Journal of Psychopharmacology 30:1181–1197.

Griffiths RR, Johnson MW, Richards WA, et al. (2018) Psilocybin-occasioned mystical-type experience in combination with meditation and other spiritual practices produces enduring positive changes in psychological functioning and in trait measures of prosocial attitudes and behaviors. Journal of Psychopharmacology 32:49–69.

Gunther M (2020) No, Richard Nixon did not call Timothy Leary 'the most dangerous man in America. Medium.

Halpern JH (2004) Hallucinogens and dissociative agents naturally growing in the United States. Pharmacology and Therapeutics 102:131–138.

Halpern JH, Pope Jr HG (2003) Hallucinogen persisting perception disorder: what do we know after 50 years? Drug and Alcohol Dependence 2003:109–119.

Hermle L, Fünfgeld M, Oepen G, et al. (1992) Mescaline-induced psychopathological, neuropsychological, and neurometabolic effects in normal subjects: experimental psychosis as a tool for psychiatric research. Biological Psychiatry 32:976–991.

Hermle L, Gouzoulis-Mayfrank E, Spitzer M (1998) Blood flow and cerebral laterality in the mescaline model of psychosis. Pharmacopsychiatry 31(S 2):85–91.

Hofmann A, Ott J (1980) LSD: my problem child. Psychedelic Reflections 24.

Hogan E (2017) Turn on, tune in, drop by the office. 1843 Magazine. The Economist Group).

Holze F, Caluori TV, Vizeli P, Liechti ME (2022) Safety pharmacology of acute LSD administration in healthy subjects. Psychopharmacology 239(6):1893–1905.

Jensen SE (1962) A treatment program for alcoholics in a mental hospital. Quarterly Journal of Studies on Alcohol 23:315–320.

Johansen PØ, Krebs TS (2015) Psychedelics not linked to mental health problems or suicidal behavior: a population study. Journal of Psychopharmacology 29:270–279.

Johnson MW, Richards WA, Griffiths RR (2008) Human hallucinogen research: guidelines for safety. Journal of Psychopharmacology 22:603–620.

Johnson MW, Garcia-Romeu A, Griffiths RR (2017) Long-term follow-up of psilocybin-facilitated smoking cessation. American Journal of Drug and Alcohol Abuse 43:55–60.

Johnson MW, Griffiths RR, Hendricks PS, Henningfield JE (2018) Setting the record straight on medical psilocybin. Scientific American.

Johnson MW, Hendricks PS, Barrett FS, Griffiths RR (2019) Classic psychedelics: an integrative review of epidemiology, therapeutics, mystical experience, and brain network function. Pharmacology and Therapeutics 197:83–102.

Khan I (1979) Convention on psychotropic substances, 1971: the role and responsibilities of the World Health Organization. Progress in Neuro-Psychopharmacology 3:11–14.

Lea T, Amada N, Jungaberle H (2020) Psychedelic microdosing: a subreddit analysis. Journal of Psychoactive Drugs 52:101–112.

Liester MB (2014) A review of lysergic acid diethylamide (LSD) in the treatment of addictions: historical perspectives and future prospects. Current Drug Abuse Reviews 7:146–156.

LoBianco T (2016) Report: aide says Nixon's war on drugs targeted blacks, hippies. CNN Politics.

McKenna T (1999) Food of the gods: the search for the original tree of knowledge: a radical history of plants, drugs and human evolution. Random House.

Minutaglio B, Davis SL (2018) The most dangerous man in America: Timothy Leary, Richard Nixon and the hunt for the fugitive king of LSD. Twelve.

Multidisciplinary Association for Psychedelic Studies (2007) The medical history of psychedelic drugs. University of Cambridge.

Nichols DE (2016) Psychedelics. Pharmacological Reviews 68:264–355.

Nichols DE, Grob CS (2018) Is LSD toxic? Forensic Science International 284:141–145.

Nichols DE, Walter H (2020) The history of psychedelics in psychiatry. Pharmacopsychiatry 54:151–166.

Nutt DJ (2019) Psychedelic drugs—a new era in psychiatry? Dialogues in Clinical Neuroscience 21:139.

Nutt DJ, King LA, Nichols DE (2013) Effects of Schedule I drug laws on neuroscience research and treatment innovation. Nature Reviews Neuroscience 14:577–585.

Nutt DJ, Erritzoe D, Carhart-Harris R (2020) Psychedelic psychiatry's brave new world. Cell 181:24–28.

Nutt DJ, Carhart-Harris R (2021) The current status of psychedelics in psychiatry. JAMA Psychiatry 78:121–122.

Orsolini L, Papanti GD, De Berardis D, et al. (2017) The 'endless trip' among the NPS users: psychopathology and psychopharmacology in the hallucinogen-persisting perception disorder. A systematic review. Frontiers in Psychiatry 8:240.

Osmond H (1957) A review of the clinical effects of psychotomimetic agents. Ann New York Academy of Sciences 66:418–434.

Reynolds HT, Vijayakumar V, Gluck-Thaler E, et al. (2018) Horizontal gene cluster transfer increased hallucinogenic mushroom diversity. Evolution Letters 2:88–101.

Robbins E, Robbins L, Frosch WA, Stern M (1967) Implications of untoward reactions to hallucinogens. Bulletin of the New York Academy of Medicine 43:985.

Roseman L, Leech R, Feilding A, et al. (2014) The effects of psilocybin and MDMA on between-network resting state functional connectivity in healthy volunteers. Frontiers in Human Neuroscience 8:204.

Ross S, Bossis A, Guss J, et al. (2016) Rapid and sustained symptom reduction following psilocybin treatment for anxiety and depression in patients with life-threatening cancer: a randomized controlled trial. Journal of Psychopharmacology 30:1165–1180.

Rucker JJ (2015) Psychedelic drugs should be legally reclassified so that researchers can investigate their therapeutic potential. BMJ 350:h2902.

Rucker JJ, Jelen LA, Flynn S, et al. (2016) Psychedelics in the treatment of unipolar mood disorders: a systematic review. Journal of Psychopharmacology 30:1220e1229.

Rucker JJ, Iliff J, Nutt DJ (2018) Psychiatry & the psychedelic drugs: past, present & future. Neuropharmacology 142:200–218.

Samorini G (1992) The oldest representations of hallucinogenic mushrooms in the world (Sahara Desert, 9000–7000 BP). Integration 2:69–78.

Sandison RA, Spencer AM, Whitelaw JDA (1954) The therapeutic value of lysergic acid diethylamide in mental illness. Journal of Mental Science 100:491–507.

Savage C (1952) Lysergic acid diethylamide (LSD-25) a clinical-psychological study. American Journal of Psychiatry 108:896–900.

Savage C, Savage E, Fadiman J, Harman W (1964) LSD: therapeutic effects of the psychedelic experience. Psychological Reports 14:111–120.

Schultz C (2013) Nixon prolonged Vietnam War for political gain—and Johnson knew about it, newly unclassified tapes suggest. Smithsonian Magazine.

Schunemann HJ, Fretheim A, Oxman AD (2006) Improving the use of research evidence in guideline development: 9. Grading evidence and recommendations. Health Research Policy and Systems 4:21.

Sessa B (2012) The psychedelic renaissance: reassessing the role of psychedelic drugs in 21st century psychiatry and society. Muswell Hill Press.

Shulgin A, Shulgin A (1997) TiHKAL. Transform Press.

Smart RG, Bateman K (1967) Unfavourable reactions to LSD: a review and analysis of the available case reports. Canadian Medical Association Journal 97:1214.

Strassman R (2018) Should we loosen the restrictions on psychedelics? Scientific American.

Strassman RJ, Qualls CR (1994) Dose-response study of N,N-dimethyltryptamine in humans. I. neuroendocrine, autonomic, and cardiovascular effects. Archives of General Psychiatry 51:85–97.

Studerus E, Kometer M, Hasler F, Vollenweider FX (2011) Acute, subacute and long-term subjective effects of psilocybin in healthy humans: a pooled analysis of experimental studies. Journal of psychopharmacology 25(11):1434–1452.

Sullivan W (1967) Studies conflict on LSD damage to chromosomes. New York Times, Archives.

Szalavitz M (2012) The legacy of the CIA's secret LSD experiments on America. Time Magazine.

Unknown author (1967) Mice injected with LSD bear deformed offspring. New York Times, Archives.

Unknown author (1971) LSD linked to dead youth. New York Times, Archives.

Unknown author (2019) Investors hope psychedelics are the new cannabis: are they high? The Economist, Business.

US Senate (1977) Project MKULTRA, The CIA's program of research in behavioral modification. Joint hearing before the US Senate Select Committee on Intelligence and the Subcommittee on Health and Scientific Research of the Committee on Human Resources. US Government Printing Office, Washington, DC.

Vollenweider FX, Leenders KL, Scharfetter C, et al. (1997) Positron emission tomography and fluorodeoxyglucose studies of metabolic hyperfrontality and psychopathology in the psilocybin model of psychosis. Neuropsychopharmacology 16:357–372.

Vollenweider FX, Vollenweider-Scherpenhuyzen MF, Babler A, et al. (1998) Psilocybin induces schizophrenia-like psychosis in humans via a serotonin-2 agonist action. Neuroreport 9:3897–3902.

Walsh C (2016) Psychedelics and cognitive liberty: reimagining drug policy through the prism of human rights. International Journal of Drug Policy 29:80–87.

Walter MN, Fridman EJN (Eds.) (2004) Shamanism: an encyclopedia of world beliefs, practices, and culture (Vol. 1). Abc-clio.

Wasson RG (1957) Seeking the magic mushroom. Life 42:100–120.

Wasson RG (1961) The hallucinogenic fungi of Mexico: an inquiry into the origins of the religious idea among primitive peoples. Botanical Museum Leaflets, Harvard University 19:137–162.

Wasson RG, Hofmann A, Ruck CA (2008) The road to Eleusis: unveiling the secret of the mysteries. North Atlantic Books.

Wink, M (2020) Evolution of the angiosperms and co-evolution of secondary metabolites, especially of Alkaloids. Reference series in Phytochemistry. Co-Evolution of Secondary Metabolites.

Winstock AR, Kaar S, Borschmann R (2014) Dimethyltryptamine (DMT): prevalence, user characteristics and abuse liability in a large global sample. Journal of Psychopharmacology 28:49–54.

Yockey RA, Vidourek RA, King KA (2020) Trends in LSD use among US adults: 2015–2018. Drug and Alcohol Dependence 212:108071.

CHAPTER 2

The psychotherapeutic component of psychedelic medicine

Laurie Higbed and Ben Sessa

KEY POINTS

- Psychedelic-assisted psychotherapy (PAP) allows therapists to embrace an individualized formulation-driven rather than a reductionist diagnostic-focused understanding of mental distress.
- PAP provides a potential alternative to long-term maintenance medications for a number of mental health problems.
- PAP offers a truly holistic approach to treatment in which a drug-induced neurological state is used purposefully to facilitate exploration of potential underlying causes of distress.
- Key therapeutic phases encompass preparation, psychedelic drug–assisted experiential sessions and post-drug integration.

Introduction

For many decades, pharmaceutical drugs such as selective serotonin reuptake inhibitors (SSRIs) have typically been a first-line pharmacological treatment offered to patients with various mental health problems including depression, eating disorders and anxiety-based disorders, including posttraumatic stress (PTSD). Whilst there is certainly a place for short-term prescribing of SSRIs in some severe psychiatric conditions, the relative efficacy of pharmacological treatment with SSRIs is poor for many patients, with a significant number of people achieving only partial or no benefit at all from medication (Frazzetto, 2008). For those who do find relief of symptoms via pharmaceutical options, the patient must rely on a daily maintenance regimen to maintain benefit. Furthermore, there is a current epidemic of over-prescribing of SSRIs—especially at the level of primary care—where the drugs are frequently inappropriately prescribed to cases of only mild to moderate depression and anxiety, and for beyond the effective length of recommended treatment, despite persisting poor outcomes (Read et al., 2021).

The fact that medications are not universally effective indicates that mental distress cannot be entirely explained by a biological model of disruption in brain chemistry. Rather, each of us has a personal narrative of complex and interwoven biological, psychological, and social factors that influence our view of ourselves, the world, people around us, and how we respond to them. This understanding of the human experience has been informed by several viewpoints over time, such as the biopsychosocial model (Engel, 1977), Relational Frame Theory (Hayes, 2004), and, more recently, the 'Power, Threat, Meaning' framework (Johnstone & Boyle, 2018). The Power, Threat, Meaning framework highlights that meaning-making and a sense of personal control are informed by individual factors (e.g. a person's beliefs, language, higher cognitions, emotions, and bodily sensations) and by systemic factors (e.g. social, economic, and relational). For example, difficult early attachment relationships, growing up in poverty, belonging to a marginalized group, having personal experience of trauma, or an early caregiver experience of incarceration and experiencing discrimination are just a few of the many causal factors identified in many mental health presentations. And, from a positive thera-peutic standpoint, because multiple varying risk factors interact together to form the eventual end phenotype, similarly, there are multiple opportunities for thera-peutic interventions across of all of these modalities. In this context, this chapter outlines the way in which psychedelic-assisted psychotherapy (PAP) can facilitate an individualized formulation-driven rather than a reductionist diagnostic-focused understanding of mental distress and help address these underlying issues.

Talking therapy treatments

Talking therapies offer the opportunity to integrate the psycho-social elements of the biopsychosocial model and allow for a formulation-driven approach of treatment, in which interventions are guided by a collaborative and holistic under-standing of the factors that have contributed to individuals' difficulties, what may be keeping them going, and any strengths and assets that they can draw from.

Specific talking therapies such as cognitive-behavioural therapy, behavioural activation, and interpersonal psychotherapy (IPT) are NICE recommended treatments in the UK and can be offered in combination with medication. The UK government's 2008 plan to increase access to psychological therapies for common mental health problems has enabled clinical populations to engage with talking therapy alongside or instead of pharmacological options. This has been emulated in other jurisdictions around the world.

However, despite this effort to increase engagement with psychological inter-ventions, talking therapies are not a panacea. People can struggle to engage with the onerous and often emotionally draining therapy process. In cases of PTSD, for example, drop-out rates from therapy are particularly high, and positive therapeutic outcomes are especially low, with rates of treatment resistance up to 50%, as some individuals find that they struggle with the overwhelming internal sensations triggered by thinking and talking about their traumatic experiences. And the rates for positive outcomes in treating addictions are even more limited, with around 75% of people relapsing after current typical treatment protocols (Moos & Moos, 2006).

Combining psychedelics with therapy: enhancing healing potential

Compounds with psychedelic properties (including LSD, psilocybin, DMT, MDMA, and ketamine) offer a very different application of pharmacological treatment as, in stark comparison to the daily maintenance treatment of SSRIs, they are typically used in protocols in which the compound is offered sparingly (usually on only two or three occasions) in combination with non-drug-assisted sessions.

Thus, pharmacological effects and psychotherapeutic processes are intentionally entwined—with these so-called mind-manifesting medicines (see Chapter 1) offering increased opportunity for increased creativity, self-exploration, and new and profound meaning-making (Groff, 2008; Hartogsohn, 2018, Watts et al., 2017). The drug-induced sessions occur within a context of careful preparation psychotherapy sessions and crucial post-drug sessions to integrate the psychedelic experience by exploring and building upon any new insights and perspectives with the support of a therapist.

This offers a truly holistic approach to treatment in which a drug-induced neurological state is used purposefully to facilitate exploration of potential underlying causes of distress. In addition, the enhanced brain plasticity (connectivity within and between brain regions) afforded by these medicines offers a prime window of opportunity to make crucial therapeutic gains that may not be achieved, or may take considerably longer, in standard treatments (Lepow et al., 2021). Furthermore, given that childhood trauma and/or adversity is well-recognized as a central causal factor for mental distress, a psychedelic-assisted therapeutic intervention can be seen as transcending diagnostic categories and facilitating a person-centred and formulation-driven approach to treatment.

What are the important factors in psychedelic-assisted psychotherapy?

The psychotherapeutic component of psychedelic medicine in modern research studies has drawn from a variety of models, including transpersonal (Grof, 2008), con-joint couples therapy (Wagner et al., 2019), Motivational Enhancement Therapy (Bogenschutz et al., 2015), and Acceptance and Commitment Therapy (Sloshower et al., 2020). Despite this variation, the core foundations of PAPs are the phases of preparation and the drug-assisted sessions themselves, followed by the opportunity to integrate the experience in a way that feels meaningful and translates into behavioural change.

Preparation

Careful preparation is crucial to allow the patients to feel able to trust themselves, the drug, and their therapist(s) during the drug-assisted sessions (Box 2.1). The

---

Box 2.1 Key elements of preparation sessions

- Creation of a safe, comfortable, and supportive environment
- Opportunity to discuss any queries and concerns, including how the medicine works in the brain and safety aspects of the medicine
- Anticipated medicine effects (physical and psychological) and expected duration
- Discussion of logistics of the dosing day
- Patient expectations (ensuring these are realistic) and their intention for the medicine-assisted session
- Familiarization with the dosing room and the default position (reclining with eyeshades and headphones with music playing)
- Concept of all experiences being welcome and providing an opportunity for healing
- Discussion and practice of how the patient may ask for support to help them to stay with internal experiences as much as they can
- Agreed boundaries on whether supportive touch is used, how it is used, and how the patient can stop touch at any time

---

well-prepared patient can go towards and be with whatever internal experiences show up as the process develops. The ability to do this offers powerful therapeutic potential; as people are given an opportunity, perhaps for the first time, to engage with and process internal experiences (this could be memories, images, physical sensations, thoughts, and emotions) without avoidance.

The mindset of patients going into their psychedelic-assisted session can have a crucial bearing on their subjective experience, thus adequate preparation with their therapist facilitates a mindset that is more likely to enhance rather than impede the drug-assisted session. The concept of 'set' refers to the internal aspect, or mindset, of the persons undergoing a psychedelic experience such as their personality, mood, intentions, and expectations (Metzer & Leary, 1967). Preparation sessions provide an opportunity for the therapist and individual to build rapport. They begin to develop a collaborative understanding of their reasons for seeking support at this time, and work together towards understanding the patient's hopes, expectations, and goals for therapy. It is important for therapists to help manage patient expectations. Most patients will have already tried many other traditional treatment options prior to discovering psychedelic therapies. These traditional approaches will often have been unhelpful or lacking in efficacy, and patients may thus be pinning their hopes of recovery on what they have heard is a potentially revolutionary alternative. Even though research using psychedelics to support the therapeutic process is extremely encouraging, there is more work to be done, and, like other treatments, it does not work for everyone. It is crucial that patients are aware of this so that expectations can be managed, and they do not risk further mental suffering if they do not benefit or if the benefits of psychedelic therapy are short-lived (see Chapter 11).

Longitudinal factors that may have influenced the patient's difficulties (including early childhood and attachment experiences, coping styles, general temperament, and key life events) are valuable to discuss in preparation as they are likely to be highly relevant to the dosing session and for the therapeutic process as a whole. For example, a key life event that has caused distress for the individual may be likely to come up spontaneously or, if deemed to be relevant to the formulation, it may be agreed during preparation that the therapist will prompt the patient during the dosing session if it does not come up naturally. Furthermore, the patient's propensity to certain coping styles can offer insights into how they may cope when faced with potentially challenging internal experiences, some of which may be more helpful than others. For example, if a patient is identified as tending to avoid emotions by intellectualizing his experience, the therapist may support him to practice noticing and 'being with' internal experiences during preparation, with a view to facilitating his ability to being open to 'collecting experiences' (Johnson et al., 2008) as best he can during the dosing day, thus offering greater healing potential.

How the patients may 'stay with' challenging material during dosing in a way that feels psychologically safe, and any support the therapist can offer to help them to do this, is explicitly discussed and practised during preparation. This may involve the use of the breath, verbal prompts, and supportive touch. If the patient agrees that touch may be beneficial, boundaries of how this is used and how the patient can stop the touch are also practised.

Patients are encouraged to bring a 'beginners mind' to the experience as much as possible (Mithoefer et al., 2017). In the MAPS manual for MDMA-assisted therapy for PTSD, Mithoefer and colleagues describe the utility of setting an intention during the preparation phase so that the patient has an idea of what they would like to gain from their dosing session, but to 'hold the intentions lightly'. If the patient (or therapist) attempts to assert too much control over the focus and content of the session, this could be counterproductive. Being open to whatever experiences naturally unfold offers the most potential for inner healing.

The preparation phase also considers the setting in which the psychedelic experience takes place. In an altered state of consciousness where suggestibility is increased and meaning-making heightened, an environment which feels comfortable, aesthetically pleasing, and not overly clinical can help to reduce the probability of psychological distress (Johnson et al., 2008). Thus, a quiet and calm space more aligned to the look of a comfortable living room than a hospital clinic is adopted with the use of cushions, blankets, plants, and low lighting.

During preparation, the patient will be introduced to and have the opportunity to practice the 'default position'; they will be encouraged to spend much of the time during dosing in a comfortable, typically reclining position, listening to music through headphones and wearing eyeshades in order to encourage and enhance an internal focus, without external distraction. This is often referred to as being 'inside'. Music is a well-established feature of psychedelic-assisted therapies and is described by Kalean et al. (2018) as 'the hidden therapist' because of its potential to affect the individual's internal experience in meaningful ways whilst under the influence of a mind-altering compound. Therapy playlists are typically carefully selected to reflect the arc of the individual's drug experience with the aim of supporting the internal healing process.

Another important aspect of the preparation sessions is psychoeducation for the patient about the drug itself. Most patients will have heard about the drug only in the context of its recreational use. Much media reporting of psychedelics is negatively biased towards harm and illegality concerns. Patients are often interested to learn about the brain mechanisms of how psychedelic drugs work and, especially, how the psychedelic drugs, when used clinically, under careful medical supervision, have a far lower risk profile than typically reported in the popular media in the context of nonclinical uses, often with erroneous conflations between recreational and clinical uses (Sessa et al., 2022).

Drug-assisted session

Classic psychedelics (such as LSD and psilocybin) and entactogens such as MDMA are relatively long-acting compared to typical psychotherapeutic clinical interventions (Box 2.2). A dosing session with psilocybin or MDMA can last at least six hours. To ensure that the patient is never alone during the experience, a two-therapist dyadic pair model is usual. To ensure sufficient rapport is gained and trust is built between the patient and both therapists, ideally both therapists will be involved in the preparation sessions prior to the psychedelic experience.

Patient safety is paramount during a dosing session. As well as conducting monitoring of physical safety, therapists aim to be as fully present as possible with the patient as the natural processing unfolds. During these sessions, interactions are most often patient-led and nondirective. The amount of time the patient spends 'inside' in the default position can vary according to compound and dose, with experiences with classic psychedelics lending themselves to an almost wholly internal focus. However, a dosing session with MDMA, with strong prosocial and anxiety-reducing effects, typically involves long periods of time spent inside interspersed with patient-led discussion with the therapists (Mithoefer et al., 2017).

Box 2.2 Key elements of drug-assisted sessions

- Therapists are ensuring safety and comfort, providing an empathic presence
- Interactions are mainly patient-led and nondirective
- Patient's attention is largely directed inwards
- Use of breath and body awareness to help patient to stay with internal experiences
- All material as potentially relevant for healing

This patient-led focus acknowledges the potential powerful healing potential that the medicine can offer for the patient to access for themselves. Sometimes, the patient may benefit from support to stay with the experiences that unfold, as discussed above, and this is practised as much as possible during preparation. They may also wish to share some relevant material with their therapists. The content of material may be related to particular clinical issues they are addressing with the therapy: for example, MDMA therapy for alcohol use disorder may focus on aspects of a person's drinking behaviour (Sessa et al., 2021). When material is shared, therapists bring their own 'beginner's mind', remaining curious and interested, asking questions that focus on the patients' emotional (rather than intellectual) processing. This means a focus on how they are experiencing what they are describing, perhaps by noticing related emotions, imagery, and physical sensations.

Integration

The psychedelic drug experience—and indeed the entire course of psychedelic therapy comprising both drug-assisted and non-drug sessions—is only the start of the journey towards full recovery and healing (Box 2.3). Integration sessions are fundamental to allow individuals to describe for themselves their internal experiences during the drug-assisted session and make meaning from these in ways that help them to take steps towards change. Integration goes beyond just the formal sessions that take place within the therapy setting, and patients will be supported to consider how their ongoing processing can be facilitated via community networks and resources.

The first integration session typically takes place the day after the dosing session. Meeting soon after dosing acknowledges that patients may have experienced something profound, meaningful, and perhaps transcendental, and the opportunity for initial reflection on this experience supports potential meanings and insights to unfold before they are forgotten or lost.

The integration phase can be seen as fundamental for psychedelics to offer meaningful potential as medicines, as it is during the period following these

---

Box 2.3 Key elements of integration sessions

- Opportunity to discuss experiences in drug-assisted session and initial personal meanings and insights
- Awareness that this will typically be an emerging and unfolding process
- Consideration of what actions the patient can take, in line with any new perspectives and insights
- Other methods to support processing are encouraged: these may include journaling, mindfulness, meditation, and physical expressions such as yoga, breathwork, bodywork, art, dance, and exercise

> **Box 2.4** Psychological flexibility
>
> '... it's as if psychedelics coax open an oyster to reveal the precious pearl inside. However, it is subsequent experience that determines whether the oyster will remain open or close again.' (p94)
>
> Source: Watts R, Luoma JB (2020) The use of the psychological flexibility model to support psychedelic assisted therapy. *Journal of Contextual Behavioral Science* 15:92–102.

experiences that patients are likely to experience increased psychological flexibility and, subsequently to be at their most open and adaptable. According to Harris (2009) psychological flexibility refers to the ability to 'open up' to all internal experiences including the difficult ones, to 'be present' in the moment and adopt a purposeful observing self, and to 'do what matters' whereby our behaviours allow us to shape our lives in accordance with our values.

Watts and Luoma (2020) are amongst a growing number of researchers who believe in the value of applying a specific therapeutic framework to PAP to support the enhanced psychological flexibility offered by these compounds and offer optimum conditions for behavioural change and longer-term wellbeing.

The true and lasting unfurling of a well-integrated psychedelic therapy course often comes many months or years after the therapy has ended. The central goal of integration is to help the patient achieve lasting and meaningful functional change. There is emerging evidence about lasting positive personality change following psychedelic use, including increased openness (MacLean et al., 2011) and an enhanced appreciation of nature (Gandy et al., 2020).

Conclusions

Contemporary research, building on many years of Western and non-Western ceremonial practice, is seeing psychedelic therapies becoming an increasingly important and valuable asset in our toolkit for mental health treatment. Modern research protocols have rightly remained true to the centuries-long indigenous practices of offering these medicines sparingly and in specific contexts with support and guidance (see Chapter 1). With careful preparation, aftercare, and ongoing embeddedness within a patient's own network, working therapeutically with the altered state of consciousness on a limited number of occasions can facilitate new and profound insights that offer a realistic treatment alternative for those experiencing mental health problems. Given the centuries of positive work that has come before this present so-called Psychedelic Renaissance (Sessa, 2018), perhaps the greatest challenge for the future of psychedelic therapies will not only be further evidencing of safety and efficacy of the treatments themselves, but rather developing meaningful large-scale applications and accessibility for public health systems (see Chapter 11). We may not be looking only at a renaissance of psychedelics, but a major renaissance of mental health care itself.

REFERENCES

Bogenschutz MP, Forcehimes AA, Pommy JA, et al. (2015) Psilocybin-assisted treatment for alcohol dependence: a proof-of-concept study. Journal of Psychopharmacology **29**:289–299.

Engel GL (1977) The need for a new medical model: a challenge for biomedicine. Science **196**:129–136.

Frazzetto G (2008) The drugs don't work for everyone: doubts about the efficacy of antidepressants renew debates over the medicalization of common distress. EMBO Reports **9**:605–608.

Gandy S, Forstmann M, Carhart-Harris RL, Timmermann C, Luke D, Watts R (2020) The potential synergistic effects between psychedelic administration and nature contact for the improvement of mental health. Health Psychology Open **7**(2).

Grof S (2008) LSD psychotherapy (4th edition): the healing potential of psychedelic medicine. Multidisciplinary Association for Psychedelic Studies.

Harris R (2009) ACT made simple: an easy-to-read primer on acceptance and commitment therapy. New Harbinger.

Hartogsohn I (2018) The meaning-enhancing properties of psychedelics and their mediator role in psychedelic therapy, spirituality, and creativity. Frontiers in Neuroscience **12**:129.

Hayes SC (2004) Acceptance and commitment therapy, relational frame theory, and the third wave of behavioral and cognitive therapies. Behavior Therapy **35**:639–665.

Johnson M, Richards W, Griffiths R (2008) Human hallucinogen research: guidelines for safety. Journal of Psychopharmacology **22**:603–620.

Johnstone L, Boyle M (2018) The power threat meaning framework: an alternative nondiagnostic conceptual system. Journal of Humanistic Psychology. https://doi.org/10.1177/0022167818793289

Kaelen M, Giribaldi B, Raine J, et al. (2018) The hidden therapist: evidence for a central role of music in psychedelic therapy. Psychopharmacology **235**:505–519.

Lepow L, Morishita H, Yehuda R (2021) Critical period plasticity as a framework for psychedelic-assisted psychotherapy. Frontiers in Neuroscience **15**:710004.

MacLean KA, Johnson MW, Griffiths RR (2011) Mystical experiences occasioned by the hallucinogen psilocybin led to increases in the personality domain of openness. Journal of Psychopharmacology **25**:1453–1461.

Metzner R, Leary T (1967) On programming psychedelic experiences. Psychedelic Review **9**:5–19.

Mithoefer M, Mithoefer A, Jerome L, et al. (2017) A manual for MDMA-assisted psychotherapy in the treatment of posttraumatic stress disorder. Retrieved from: https://s3-us-west-1.amazonaws.com/mapscontent/research-archive/mdma/TreatmentManual_MDMAAssistedPsychotherapyVersion+8.1_22+Aug2017.pdf.

Moos RH, Moos BS (2006) Rates and predictors of relapse after natural and treated remission from alcohol use disorders. Addiction 101:212–222.

Read J, Cartwright C, Gibson K (2021) Are antidepressants overprescribed? Patients' experiences of the prescribing process. Ethical Human Psychology and Psychiatry 22:83–97.

Sessa B (2018) The 21st century psychedelic renaissance: heroic steps forward on the back of an elephant. Psychopharmacology 235:551–560.

Sessa B, Higbed L, O'Brien S, et al. (2021) First study of safety and tolerability of 3,4-methylenedioxymethamphetamine-assisted psychotherapy in patients with alcohol use disorder. Journal of Psychopharmacology 35:375–383.

Sessa B, Aday JS, O'Brien S, Curran HV, Measham F, Higbed L, Nutt DJ (2022) Debunking the myth of 'Blue Mondays': no evidence of affect drop after taking clinical MDMA. Journal of Psychopharmacology 36(3):360–367. doi:10.1177/02698811211055809. Epub 2021 Dec 13. PMID: 34894842.

Sloshower J, Guss J, Krause R (2020) The Yale manual for psilocybin-assisted therapy of depression (using acceptance and commitment therapy as a therapeutic frame). doi:10.31234/osf.io/u6v9y.

Wagner AC, Mithoefer MC, Mithoefer AT, Monson CM (2019) Combining cognitive-behavioral conjoint therapy for PTSD with 3,4-methylenedioxymethamphetamine (MDMA): a case example. Journal of Psychoactive Drugs 51:166–173.

Watts R, Day C, Krzanowski, J, et al. (2017) Patients' accounts of increased 'connectedness' and 'acceptance' after psilocybin for treatment-resistant depression. Journal of Humanistic Psychology 57:520–564.

Watts R, Luoma JB (2020) The use of the psychological flexibility model to support psychedelic assisted therapy. Journal of Contextual Behavioral Science 15:92–102.

CHAPTER 3

Psilocybin

James J. Rucker and David Erritzoe

> **KEY POINTS**
>
> - Psilocybin is a tryptamine psychedelic occurring in nature that likely has been used by people for thousands of years.
> - Psilocybin is a partial agonist of type 2A serotonin receptors in the brain, which mediates the subjective effect.
> - Psilocybin therapy has been through early phase clinical trials, but definitive trials used for medical licensing are awaited.
> - The safety and efficacy of psilocybin therapy is probably context-dependent, which challenges the interpretation of clinical trials and wider implementation if licensed.
> - If licensed, psilocybin therapy will need to be carefully regulated to ensure safety, consistency, and quality of delivery.

Introduction

Psilocybin is a tryptamine molecule found in a broad range of mushroom species that grow throughout the world. As detailed in Chapter 1, historical evidence for the use of psilocybin-containing mushrooms suggests ritualistic use by geographically dispersed cultures over millennia, continuing through to the present day. Despite fifty years of criminal sanctions in many countries for possession of psilocybin, sizable minorities of people continue to cite periodic (but not dependent) use, reporting motivations that stretch beyond recreation or hedonism. The subjective effects of psilocybin appear both challenging and rewarding, eliciting a 'dream-like' state with preserved memory formation that likely reflects an underlying disruption of the generative mechanisms of normal waking consciousness. Similar to preprohibition clinical use, modern clinical researchers have hypothesized that this state may be a useful adjunct to the wider process of psychotherapy in the treatment of a broad range of neuropsychiatric problems (see Chapter 2). Small-scale clinical trials are promising but should not be used to make judgements about wider efficacy or clinical utility. The results of larger, multicentre clinical trials will be informative. The first of these was published in November 2022, with encouraging and clinically credible results.

Psychopharmacology

Psilocybin is a broad partial agonist of serotonin (5-hydroxytryptamine; 5-HT) receptors. Psilocybin itself is not overtly psychoactive, but is rapidly metabolized to psilocin, which is. For consistency, we refer to psilocybin from now on. Like most other psychedelics, the subjective effect of psilocybin appears to be dependent on a functionally selective action on type 2A 5-HT receptors, particularly those present in layer five of the neocortex. Functional selectivity refers to the precise conformational changes in a receptor elicited by a drug. The concept is likely important because other drugs that are also agonists at 5-HT2A do not produce subjective psychedelic effects, for example lisuride.

In common with most other 5-HT receptors, 5-HT2A is a G-protein coupled receptor attached to a variety of molecular second messenger systems in the neurone that change the timing and phase of firing, control intracellular calcium homeostasis, and modulate genetic regulation of neuronal and synaptic function, possibly via the molecular target of rapamycin (mTOR) (López-Giménez & González-Maeso, 2017). Macroscopic measurements of the human brain under psychedelics using functional magnetic resonance neuroimaging (fMRI) and electroencephalographic techniques reveal decoherence of cortical network dynamics, increased spontaneous neural signal diversity (i.e. increased complexity) and suppression of cortical alpha waves, when compared with placebo. Such observations correlate well with psilocybin (specifically, psilocin) plasma concentrations, 5-HT2A receptor occupancy, and subjective intensity ratings. Increased occupancy of the 5-HT2A receptor, as assessed with positron emission tomography, is tightly correlated with increased intensity of subjective experience under psilocybin. Selective pharmacological blockade of the 5-HT2A receptor obviates this effect.

It is possible that there is some similarity between the mechanism of action of psilocybin and ketamine (an antagonist at N-methyl-D-aspartate (NMDA) receptors). Both appear to lead indirectly to a surge in glutamate release in areas of the prefrontal cortex that may be implicated in the pathophysiology of some neuropsychiatric illnesses: for example, major depressive disorder. However, it is unclear whether these observations have relevance to treatment or clinical response. A schematic of knowledge leading to glutamate release and modulation of second messenger systems is presented in Figure 3.1.

Psilocybin has little or absent activity on receptor systems that mediate functions such as breathing, blood pressure, or heart rhythm. Consequently, large overdoses of psilocybin-mushrooms are generally not seriously toxic to the body, and there are almost no reports of deaths from the direct effects of psilocybin. A similar picture is observed for d-lysergic acid diethylamide (LSD: see Chapter 4). Population research does not support the hypothesis that psilocybin-mushroom use is linked to the emergence of psychotic disorders, although coincident cases certainly occur. The hypothesis remains that psilocybin may 'unmask' psychosis in those with pre-existing biopsychosocial vulnerabilities.

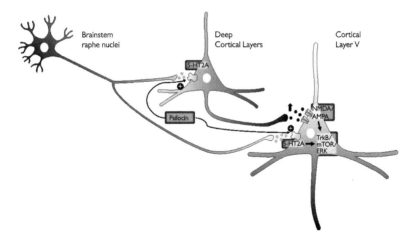

Figure 3.1 In this speculative model, direct stimulation of 5-HT2A, as well as indirect stimulation of NMDA/AMPA, receptors by psilocin may converge on intracellular mechanisms implicated in neuronal plasticity and synapse regulation that may underpin antidepressant effects.

Effects on the brain

Psilocybin elicits a subjective state described succinctly as 'a waking dream'. Unlike dreams, memory formation and insight usually remain intact. Like dreams, the nature and range of consciously experienced mental processes is broad and shifted towards 'imprecision' relative to normal waking consciousness. Sensory distortions, strong emotions, phantasmagoria, and blurring of conceptual boundaries are, therefore, common and dose dependent.

As discussed in Chapter 11, the subjective state is often probed with visual analogue scales such as the Altered State of Consciousness questionnaire. 'Bliss', 'elemental imagery', 'experience of unity', 'spiritual experience', 'insightfulness', and 'audiovisual synaesthesia' are reliably more highly rated under psilocybin than comparator conditions. However, since psilocybin may also be understood as a nonspecific 'amplifier' of mental processes, the range and degree of reported experiences also includes negative experiences such as panic, paranoia, and frank hallucinations.

The effects of psilocybin seem in part dependent on the mind 'set' of the individual, as well as the 'setting' in which the drug is given, perhaps more so than other drugs. Given the position of the 5-HT2A receptor in the neocortex, it is reasonable to hypothesize that psychedelics modulate the cognitive mechanisms that govern expectation formation and suggestibility, although the relative role of the 5-HT2A receptor is doubtless part of an exceptionally complex system. This is illustrated, relative to the proposed action of serotonergic reuptake inhibitor antidepressants, in Figure 3.2a,b.

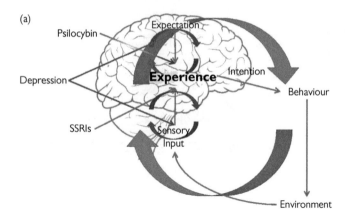

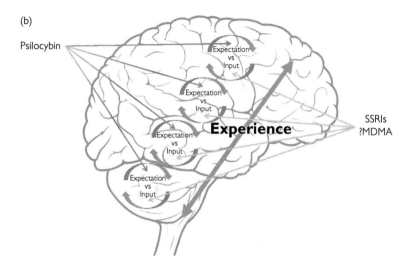

Figure 3.2 (a) In this simplified, speculative model, psilocybin is proposed to modify expectations of sensory input, whereas serotonergic reuptake inhibitor drugs are proposed to modify the afffective valence attached to sensory input itself. (b) Continuing from 3.2a, the nature and content of experience is considered as part of multi-dimensional, hierarchal 'competition' between different sensory domains, where psilocybin predominantly modulates expectation, and SSRIs/MDMA predominantly modulate the valence of incoming sensory experience. Depending on the nature of a given mental health problem, either (or both) interventions may have value.

This brings into play a more nuanced discussion of the role that psychedelics: such as, psilocybin may have in moderating the placebo response within different psychotherapeutic paradigms. In this sense, it is interesting to consider whether psilocybin and related compounds might be forms of pharmacologically active 'super-placebos' within a wider psychotherapeutic milieu. Observations from the clinical use of LSD and mescaline prior to prohibition in 1970 support the notion that the psychedelics served as 'catalysts' of change in those already engaged in psychotherapy and who were motivated to improve. Such theories are challenging for existing paradigms of clinical trial design and outcome measurement in psychiatry to accommodate. These issues are discussed further below, and in Chapter 11.

Clinical trials

Clinical trials with psilocybin resumed in 1996 with the publication of phase 1, first-in-human pharmacokinetic and safety studies in healthy volunteers. Peak plasma concentrations of psilocin occur approximately 100 minutes after oral administration of psilocybin, and the half-life of psilocin is approximately 163 minutes. Clinically significant psychoactive effects are reported with plasma concentrations above 4 ng/ml. No serious adverse events were reported in these studies, and psilocybin was generally well tolerated, with a repertoire of generally 'expected' psychedelic effects that also included occasional negative experiences of dysphoria and anxiety. These are summarized comprehensively elsewhere (Studerus et al., 2011).

The largest clinical trial in healthy volunteers up to 2021 took place in the UK in 2019 (Rucker et al., 2022). Eighty-nine participants were randomly assigned to receive a single dose of placebo, 10 mg or 25 mg of psilocybin in a clinical research environment under double blind conditions (although the effectiveness of blinding was not further assessed). Up to six participants were dosed simultaneously. Total follow-up was for three months. The primary objective was to assess the effects of psilocybin on emotional processing and cognitive function at one week and four weeks after dosing.

Cognitive and emotional function assessments showed no clinically relevant short- or long-term negative effect of psilocybin at either the 10 mg or 25 mg doses, compared to placebo at either one- or four-week follow-up. There were no significant differences between psilocybin-naïve and psilocybin experienced participants. The 10 mg and 25 mg doses of psilocybin were generally well tolerated, with most treatment-emergent adverse events being of mild or moderate severity. There were no treatment-emergent serious adverse events (SAEs) and no adverse events that led to study withdrawal.

Published clinical trials with psilocybin in patients conducted between 2006 and 2021 are summarized in Table 3.1. Most trials have been open-label pilot and feasibility randomized controlled trials that are primarily designed to probe safety rather than efficacy. The first trial—in 2006—involved nine patients with

Table 3.1 Published clinical trials with psilocybin therapy in patients—conducted between 2006 and 2021

Study	Year	Treatment Population	Design	Subjects (N)	Dose(s)	Number of Dosing Sessions	Duration of Follow-Up	Therapy Model	Outcomes
Moreno et al., 2006	2006	Obsessive compulsive disorder	Phase 1b/2a Open-label, dose escalation	9	0.1 mg/kg, 0.2 mg/kg, 0.3 mg/kg	3	6 months	Not reported	≥50% decrease in Yale-Brown Obsessive-Compulsive score at 24 hours for at least 1 dose in 2/3 of participants; 11.1% reported long-term remission
Grob et al., 2011	2011	Existential distress & anxiety symptoms in life-threatening diagnoses	Phase 2a Randomized, active comparator, crossover	12	0.2 mg/kg	1	Minimum 3 months	Psychological support	Trait anxiety significantly reduced at 1- and 3-months post dosing
Johnson et al., 2014	2014	Tobacco addiction	Phase 1b/2a Open label	15	0.29 mg/kg, 0.43 mg/kg	2–3	12+ months	Addiction CBT	Abstinence rate of 67% at 12 months
Bogenschutz et al., 2015	2015	Alcohol use disorder	Phase 1b/2a Open label	10	0.3 mg/kg, 0.4 mg/kg	1–2	36 weeks	Motivational enhancement therapy	Significant reduction in heavy drinking days after first treatment, strong correlation (r = 0.76–0.89) between acute drug effects and outcomes

Study	Year	Indication	Phase/Design	N	Dose	Sessions	Support	Outcomes
Griffiths et al., 2016	2016	Existential distress, anxiety, & depression symptoms in life-threatening diagnoses	Phase 2a Randomized, active comparator, crossover	51	0.31 mg/kg, 0.43 mg/kg	1	6 months	Psychological support	92% response/60% remission rate at 5 weeks in treatment group vs. 32% and 16% for active placebo
Ross et al., 2016	2016	Cancer patients with depression and/or anxiety	Phase 2a Randomized, active comparator, crossover	29	0.3 mg/kg	1	6 months	Existential psychotherapy	BDI depression score: ~80% remission at 7 weeks in treatment group vs. ~10% in active placebo group, antidepressant/anxiolytic response rates 60%–80% at 6 months, outcomes correlated with subjective experience ratings
Carhart-Harris et al., 2016/2018	2016	Treatment-resistant depression	Phase 1b/2a Open label	20	10 mg, 25 mg	2	6 months	Psychological support	Significant reductions in depressive symptoms at 5 weeks (Cohen's d = 2.3), with sustained results at 6 months (Cohen's d = 1.4), outcomes correlated with subjective experience ratings

(continued)

Table 3.1 Continued

Study	Year	Treatment Population	Design	Subjects (N)	Dose(s)	Number of Dosing Sessions	Duration of Follow-Up	Therapy Model	Outcomes
Davis et al., 2020	2020	Major depressive disorder	Phase 2a Randomized, wait-list controlled	24	0.29 mg/kg, 0.43 mg/kg	2	4 weeks	Psychological support	Significant reductions in depressive symptoms at 4 weeks post treatment in immediate treatment group vs. delayed (Cohen's d = 3.3), 54% in remission 4 weeks post treatment, in immediate treatment group, improvements correlated with subjective experience ratings
Anderson et al., 2020	2020	Demoralization in HIV/AIDS	Phase 1b/2a Open label	18	0.3 mg/kg, 0.36 mg/kg	1	3 months	Brief group therapy	Clinically meaningful reduction in demoralization at 3 months (standardized effect size estimate drm = 0.97)
Schindler et al., 2020	2020	Migraine headache	Phase 2a Randomized, placebo controlled, crossover	10	0.14 mg/kg	1	3 months	Psychological support	Significant decrease in migraine frequency in treatment group for 2 weeks after treatment, no correlation between subjective effects and change in migraine frequency

Study	Year	Condition	Design	N	Dose	Sessions	Follow-up	Adjunct	Results
Carhart-Harris et al., 2021	2021	Major depression	Phase 2a Randomized, active comparator	59	25 mg	2	6 weeks	Psychological support	No significant difference in change in QIDS-SR16 scores when comparing treatment arms, 70% response & 57% remission rates in psilocybin arm vs. 57% response & 28% remission in escitalopram arm, most secondary analyses favoured psilocybin arm
Goodwin et al., 2022	2022	Treatment resistant depression	Phase 2b, randomized, dose finding	233	25 mg, 10 mg, 1 mg	1	12 weeks	Psychological support	Least-squares mean changes from baseline to week 3 in the MADRS score were −12.0 for 25 mg, −7.9 for 10 mg, and −5.4 for 1 mg; the difference between the 25-mg group and 1-mg group was −6.6 (95% confidence interval [CI], −10.2 to −2.9; P < 0.001)

obsessive compulsive disorder, who were given three doses of psilocybin in a dose-escalation design. Five years later a randomized, active-control study was published in which twelve participants with existential distress associated with life-threatening diagnoses were given a single dose of psilocybin alongside psychological support. Subsequent studies up to 2016 with similar designs have probed tobacco addiction, alcohol use disorder, and treatment-resistant depression in small numbers of patients. The nature of psychological support given was often nonspecific, ranging between a total of twelve and eighteen hours per participant. No SAEs were reported. Nausea, anxiety, fatigue, and headache were reported in over 20% of participants. Transient rises in heart rate and blood pressure (usually not deemed to be of clinical significance) were not uncommon. Psychotic-like symptoms were not seen lasting beyond the acute effects of the drug. Overall, these trials have not identified clinically concerning safety signals.

In a head to head design, fifty-nine participants with major depressive disorder in a single centre in the UK were randomised to receive two sessions of 25 mg psilocybin therapy or two sessions of 1 mg psilocybin therapy, with participants receiving, respectively, placebo and 10/20 mg of escitalopram during six weeks of subsequent follow-up (Carhart-Harris et al., 2021). The primary purpose of this trial was not clinical but rather aimed to explore comparative neuroimaging mechanisms between groups (Daws et al., 2022). The main clinical efficacy outcome measure in this study was the participant rated Quick Inventory of Depressive Symptoms. This did not statistically separate between the two groups at the primary end point (three weeks after the second dosing), however the trial was not powered a priori to distinguish between groups on clinical efficacy parameters. There were no SAEs reported, and the most common adverse events in both groups were nausea and headache. Reporting on the primary neuroimaging results is discussed in Chapter 11 (Daws et al., 2022).

By far the largest and most rigorous study at the time of writing is a randomized, double blind study in 233 participants with carefully defined treatment-resistant depression (Goodwin et al., 2022). This study took place in twenty-two sites in ten countries across Europe and North America. Participants were randomly assigned to receive a single dose of 1 mg, 10 mg, or 25 mg of psilocybin, along with a package of psychological support, and followed up over twelve weeks. There was a highly statistically significant difference in the change in the primary outcome measure (Montgomery Asberg Depression Rating Scale) at three weeks between the 1 mg and 25 mg group, persisting until six weeks. Nearly one third of participants did not meet criteria for depression at three weeks, with one in five participants exhibiting a sustained response at twelve weeks. The most frequent adverse events were headache, nausea and dizziness. Suicidal or self injury behaviour was observed in three participants in the 25mg group, however all were non-responders at week three.

In other indications, a recent trial of patients ($n = 93$) with alcohol use disorder randomly assigned participants to two doses of psilocybin or the antihistamine diphenhydramine; all participants also received psychological support, including motivational interviewing and cognitive behaviour therapy (Bogenschutz et al., 2022). There was a significant difference between the study arms on the primary outcome measure, namely heavy drinking days (at thirty-two-week follow-up, psilocybin patients had a mean of 9.7% versus 23.6% for diphenhydramine; standard mean difference 13.9%; 95%CI 3.0–24.7). In this trial, 93.6% of participants correctly guessed their treatment allocation in session one, with a mean certainty of 88.5%. In the second session, 94.7% correctly guessed their allocation, with a mean certainty of 90.6%. Study therapists correctly guessed allocation 92.4% of the time in the first session, and 97.4% in the second session. Numerous other trials are in progress or planning (see Chapter 11).

As discussed in Chapter 11, clinical trials with psilocybin are often criticized for insufficiently controlling for placebo or expectancy effects. As has been shown, it is not possible to blind participants to allocation in psilocybin therapy trials. Expectancy effects are unavoidable. Blinding procedures are nonetheless employed, including allocation concealment and blinded independent ratings of the primary outcome. It is hard to envisage what else is practical or useful. Some have suggested that the adequacy of blinding should be measured routinely. This is possible, but the result is likely to be much argument about 'what is drug and what is expectancy', when the distinction may be clinically meaningless anyway (see below). Similar issues exist in trials of surgical procedures, physiotherapy, and psychotherapy, but few question the place of these interventions in healthcare.

The peculiarity of attempting to account for expectancy effects in psilocybin therapy trials is that psilocybin is likely to affect the cognitive mechanism of expectancy effects themselves. If so, then to account for them makes little logical sense. Users of psychedelics are known to be more suggestible whilst under their influence, rendered 'sensitive to context'. Thus, context will moderate outcome and this is unavoidable. This may have much clinical relevance, but it challenges established paradigms of trial design that attempt to separate treatments from their contexts. Thus, we need to be clear what questions clinical trials with psilocybin therapy can realistically answer. They will likely answer questions about relative safety well. Questions about efficacy and effectiveness will be open to argument. Questions about the nature and degree of expectancy effects are unlikely to be answered with much satisfaction at all. More useful directions might be explorations of the elements of context that are positive or negative moderators of outcome for most people. Here, many things seem self-evident, but qualitative analysis may help to pick out consistent, clinically useful themes. This may have relevance well beyond psilocybin therapy.

Delivery of clinical trials with psilocybin

Medical psilocybin is not yet available for clinical use outside of government approved clinical trials. As of March 2022, no regulatory approval exists for any indication and clinical trials are ongoing. A variety of clinical and regulatory issues surround the research use of psilocybin.

Psilocybin is generally placed in the most restrictive categories of international and national drug regulation statutes. This usually means that manufacturers, hospitals, academic institutions, and prescribing clinicians require special government licenses to handle psilocybin, complying with high burdens of security and safe custody. This limitation has prevented many institutions from undertaking research with psilocybin.

Psilocybin remains legally stigmatized as a 'dangerous drug of abuse'. Whilst this is scientifically unsound, such stigma permeates through the layers of governance and implementation around clinical trials and medical use. This likely has a myriad of effects. On the one hand, approvals for psilocybin trials may be denied on grounds of safety, particularly when reviewed by those unfamiliar with the drugs or the safeguards used in the research. On the other hand, trials may be authorized on the grounds of 'challenging the mistakes of history', risking distraction from patient safety concerns. Those who volunteer for such trials may bring similarly polarized views. Significant expectation can be placed on a single psilocybin therapy treatment, when the reality is that the chance of a life changing experience is limited. Both positive and negative expectancy can be amplified by team dynamics, the environment of dosing, therapist relationships, and personal preferences about music and décor, as well as by the day-to-day stresses and strains that may accompany participants and therapists into the dosing room. Introducing psilocybin into this milieu is, inherently, a gamble.

A culture of trust, transparency, learning, and mutual respect seem fundamental to mitigate some of the risks inherent in this. The infrastructure surrounding a clinical trial with psilocybin needs to be sufficiently robust to support a study team comfortably, without exerting unnecessary bureaucratic pressure. Similarly, a study team needs to be sufficiently expert and cohesive to recruit appropriate participants and 'hold' over time the emotional distress that mentally unwell participants bring. This demands a certain 'slack in the system' that efficiency-hungry managerialism can be reluctant to accommodate. Study teams need to be sufficiently committed to 'go the extra mile' when required. However, this needs to be balanced by clear boundaries and definitions about the limits of practical and emotional support that the team can deliver. Taken together, this should help to manage expectations appropriately, safeguard participants, and reduce the risk of unprofessional behaviour. Only with all of this in place can a proper therapeutic space be created that allows the process of treatment to take place between therapists and participants. Consistent, compassionate, and ethical models of leadership and supervision are likely the containers that allow this wider process to occur and accrue, bringing back into focus the overall culture, values, and supervisory structures of the institutions that host the trials.

The setting for psilocybin dosing has been covered extensively elsewhere, including in Chapter 2 of this book. It should be quiet and comfortable. Psilocybin is notably nontoxic to body systems, thus the likelihood of need for acute or emergency medical care is low (but not zero). An emerging model of therapy delivery emphasizes core competencies of trust-building, psychoeducation, nonjudgmental emotional support, active listening, and a flexible (yet boundaried) approach that can adjust to the diagnosis, participant narratives, and therapist-participant dynamics as they evolve. The intended outcome is a more positive and proactive perspective on the precipitating and perpetuating problems that contribute to poor mental health, which in turn serve as a foundation for longer term, sustainable improvements in functioning.

Trial 'aftercare' can be problematic. Ethics committees often insist on defined transfers of care between researchers and referrers, after which a trial team should not be providing day-to-day care. Similarly, trial funders generally will not fund interventions beyond the last visit. This can lead to participants feeling bereft and let down when the nuanced care of the trial team ends. Public-facing integration groups can ease this transition. Here, the model is peer support, moderated by those experienced with group therapy principles.

Future prospects & problems

The latest results from multicentre phase 2b trials of psilocybin therapy for treatment-resistant depression pave the way for phase 3 clinical trials, due to start in late 2022. In this sense, the pathway to medical licensing of psilocybin therapy (for this indication) is clear.

And yet there are obvious and unusual challenges to the clinical trials paradigm of treatment development. Here, psilocybin therapy does not fit easily. There may be regulatory confusion about how to license and regulate it. Medicines regulatory bodies (FDA in the United States, EMA in Europe, and the MHRA in the UK, for example) are likely to want to treat psilocybin the same as any other drug, even though this is only one part of the treatment. Beyond this, it seems obvious that the psychological support package and context of delivery will need to be regulated to ensure they are delivered in a consistent and quality assured way.

If approved, the delivery of psilocybin therapy is likely to be expensive and logistically complicated compared to existing generic drug therapies and short-term or online psychotherapy interventions. On the other hand, it is likely to be less expensive than specialised treatments such as long term psychotherapy, electroconvulsive therapy and inpatient admission. It may be similar in cost to ketamine therapy, now increasingly a standard form of treatment for resistant depression in secondary care. Health economic analyses are underway.

If someone is willing to pay, then facilities will need to be available. Psilocybin therapy is not a medically complicated intervention to deliver, thus it is likely that existing mental healthcare infrastructure will be suitable with some cosmetic modification. Progress is already being made in various centres in the United States and Europe to explore this, and the recent delivery of clinics delivering ketamine treatment sets a precedent.

Finally, allegations of abuse, misconduct, and cover-up in underground psychedelic 'therapy' sessions are very concerning. This raises the issue of whether they could be repeated in clinical trials or in licensed use. This is certainly possible.

However, medical regulation comes with legally enforceable obligations around ethical and professional conduct; the absolute requirement for documented, informed consent; and established routes for safeguarding and monitoring of therapeutic provision. Whilst these processes cannot absolutely prevent such abuses from occurring, they should serve as a framework to reduce the risk. Discrete video monitoring of psilocybin therapy sessions seems a logical step to further reassure, a step which is already undertaken in many psilocybin therapy trials.

Conclusions

Psilocybin has a unique and special history. Its pharmacology lends itself to paradigms of drug-assisted therapy, paradigms that were explored within medical and psychotherapeutic contexts prior to legal prohibition around 1970. The contemporary medical development of psilocybin therapy for treatment-resistant depression now has significant momentum. This said, licensing is by no means inevitable, and definitive trials are awaited. There are challenges inherent to clinical trials with psilocybin therapy, psilocybin therapy itself, and the wider context of the effects of stigma and prohibition. It remains to be seen whether these challenges can be dealt with in a manner that garners the wider support of regulators, healthcare practitioners, and the public. However, the current clinical trial evidence is promising.

REFERENCES

Bogenschutz MP, Ross S, Bhatt S, et al. (2022) Percentage of heavy drinking days following psilocybin-assisted psychotherapy vs placebo in the treatment of adult patients with alcohol use disorder: a randomized clinical trial. JAMA Psychiatry 79(10):953–962. doi:10.1001/jamapsychiatry.2022.2096.

Carhart-Harris R, Giribaldi B, Watts R, et al. (2021) Trial of psilocybin versus escitalopram for depression. New England Journal of Medicine **384**:1402–1411.

Daws R, Timmermann C, Giribaldi B, et al. (2022) Increased global integration in the brain after psilocybin therapy for depression. Nature Medicine **28**:844–851.

Goodwin G, Aaronson, ST, Alvarez O, et al. (2022) Single-dose psilocybin for a treatment-resistant episode of major depression. New England Journal of Medicine **387**:1637–1648.

López-Giménez JF, González-Maeso J (2017) Hallucinogens and serotonin 5-HT2A receptor-mediated signaling pathways, in AL Halberstadt, FX Vollenweider, DE Nichols, ed., Behavioral neurobiology of psychedelic drugs. Springer, 45–73.

Rucker JJ, Marwood L, Ajantaival R-LJ, et al. (2022) The effects of psilocybin on cognitive and emotional functions in healthy participants: results from a phase 1, randomised, placebo-controlled trial involving simultaneous psilocybin administration and preparation. Journal of Psychopharmacology **36**:119–130.

Studerus E, Kometer M, Hasler F, Vollenweider FX (2011) Acute, subacute and long-term subjective effects of psilocybin in healthy humans: a pooled analysis of experimental studies. Journal of Psychopharmacology **25**:1434–1452.

CHAPTER 4

MDMA

Michael C. Mithoefer and David E. Presti

> **KEY POINTS**
>
> - MDMA (3,4-methylenedioxymethamphetamine) is a compound first synthesized early in the twentieth century.
> - Various names have been used to describe MDMA, including psychedelic, entheogenic, empathogenic, and entactogenic.
> - Acute central nervous system effects of MDMA are mediated primarily via enhanced release of serotonin, norepinephrine, and dopamine; oxytocin is also released.
> - Efficacy of MDMA for PTSD has been demonstrated in a number of Phase 2 trials, and a recent largescale multicentre Phase 3 trial; a confirmatory study has been completed and results are pending.
> - In clinical trials MDMA has proven to have a good safety profile.

Introduction

MDMA (3,4-methylenedioxymethamphetamine) has been variously called psychedelic, entheogenic, empathogenic, and entactogenic. While it does have mind-manifesting qualities (the etymology of the word 'psychedelic'), MDMA is very different in character from the classic psychedelics (LSD, psilocybin, DMT, and mescaline). Notably, it does not give rise to the hallucinatory activity often associated with classic psychedelics. Rather, it has the capacity to lower psychological defences, and it creates opportunities for emotional exploration, communication, and a sense of connection with one's authentic self and by extension with others. This is one of MDMA's most profound features, making it a valuable adjunct to psychotherapy and a powerful experience in other settings as well (Adamson, 2012; Greer & Tolbert, 1998; Holland, 2001). While MDMA often occasions a reduction of fear and anxiety, MDMA-assisted therapy may also be accompanied by challenging anxiety or other painful emotions. Managing this effectively requires careful preparation and integration, as well as the provision of a supportive holding environment during the MDMA-treatment sessions.

The terms 'entactogen' ('touching within') and 'empathogen' ('occasioning empathy for self and the challenges one may be experiencing, and empathy for others') have also been proposed as labels that highlight the unique qualities of MDMA (Adamson, 2012). Another drug possessing these qualities is MDMA's close chemical relative MDA (3,4-methylenedioxyamphetamine), although MDA is generally reported as more hallucinatory (Nichols, 1986).

First synthesized and patented by Merck chemical company in Germany in 1912–1914, MDMA was initially of no specific import beyond being an inter-mediate in the synthesis of another chemical in which Merck had interest. In the decades following, Merck conducted unpublished exploratory physiology studies and, in the 1950s, the US Army conducted toxicity studies in animals. Throughout this time, there is no indication of any testing in humans, or any evidence that the unique psychotropic properties of MDMA were suspected (Freudenmann et al., 2006; Holland, 2001). The chemical structure is shown in Figure 4.1.

In 1955, pharmacologist Gordon Alles (1901–1963) reported on the hallucino-genic properties of MDA (not MDMA), and during the 1960s, MDA acquired a reputation in the recreational scene as a sensual and euphorigenic 'hug and love' drug. Concurrently, MDA was explored as a psychotherapeutic agent by Claudio Naranjo (1932–2019) and by Leo Zeff (1912–1988), but legal availability of MDA ceased in 1970 when the US Controlled Substances Act classified it as Schedule 1 substance (Passie & Benzenhöfer, 2016; Passie, 2018).

Beginning in early 1960s, Alexander Shulgin (1925–2014) conducted system-atic exploration of the syntheses and psychotropic properties of novel molecules related in chemical structure to mescaline—molecules having a phenethylamine core to their structure. And in the 1970s, Shulgin received reports of interesting psychotropic properties of MDMA and set out to investigate its synthesis and properties more thoroughly (Shulgin & Nichols, 1978; Shulgin & Shulgin, 1991). He shared his observations on the human effects of MDMA with his friend the psychotherapist Leo Zeff, and Zeff, after experiencing MDMA's capacity to occasion reduced anxiety and emotional openness, spread the word in his psychotherapeutic community and educated numerous other therapists in its ad-ministration (Stolaroff, 2004).

At this time, in the 1970s and into the 1980s, therapists using MDMA in their work largely kept a low profile, not wishing to draw popular attention to MDMA and risk having it deemed illegal and unavailable. However, it proved difficult to keep such a potent emotional catalyst secret, and by the early 1980s, there was increased rec-reational use of MDMA and subsequent media attention (Grob, 2000). The name 'ecstasy' was introduced to attract customers in the uncontrolled market. Other names that have been applied to MDMA over the years are Adam, E, X, and molly.

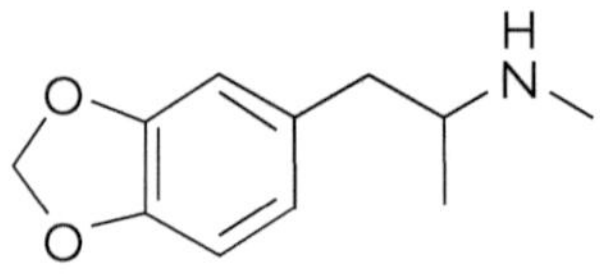

Figure 4.1 MDMA: 3,4-methylenedioxymethamphetamine.

In 1985 the US federal government invoked an emergency scheduling procedure to deem MDMA a Schedule 1 drug, making it unavailable for legal therapeutic use. At this point, therapists using MDMA began to openly discuss the success of their work (Adamson, 2012; Greer & Tolbert, 1986) and efforts were mounted to oppose the government restrictions. Some temporary success was achieved, but by 1988 the US government had overridden these efforts and MDMA was 'permanently' placed in Schedule 1, where it has remained since. Already at that point, however, a vision had formed to bring MDMA back to a place of legal availability for clinical use and further investigation.

Moving forward according to regulatory rules for drug development, in the mid-1990s Phase 1 clinical trials were conducted, establishing safety in healthy volunteers. Starting in 2004 Phase 2 and Phase 3 clinical studies followed for the treatment of posttraumatic stress disorder. A few trials for other clinical indications have also been conducted, and others are under way or in development (see Clinical trials section, below, and Chapter 11).

Neurobiology

The impacts of MDMA on the body and mind are believed to be mediated primarily via effects on neurons synthesizing and releasing the monoamine neurotransmitters serotonin, norepinephrine, and dopamine. MDMA interacts both with monoamine reuptake-transporter proteins located in axon-terminal plasma membrane and with vesicular transporters within the axon terminals, in both cases disrupting normal function (Rudnick & Wall, 1992).

Normally, plasma-membrane reuptake transporters resorb released neurotransmitter back into the presynaptic neuron. Instead, MDMA is taken up into the cell via the transporter, and in exchange neurotransmitter is now *released* via the transporter protein. In essence, the transporter no longer functions to resorb neurotransmitter, and instead functions as a releaser of neurotransmitter, a reversal of its normal role.

Vesicular monoamine transporters normally function to fill the storage vesicles with neurotransmitter, in preparation for nerve-impulse-evoked transmitter release from the cell. However, once inside the neuron, MDMA interacts with vesicular monoamine transporters and triggers *release* of neurotransmitter from the storage vesicles into the cytoplasm—again a reversal of normal function—thus making additional neurotransmitter available to exit the cell, via the MDMA-disrupted plasma-membrane transporter, into the synaptic cleft.

In short, the primary neurochemical action of MDMA is to occasion a large release of monoamine neurotransmitters and thereby enhance short-term signal activity at synapses utilizing these transmitters. The effect on release is greatest for serotonin and norepinephrine. Dopamine release is also affected, although to a lesser extent (Rothman et al., 2001).

In the peripheral nervous system, norepinephrine is the transmitter in the sympathetic branch of the autonomic system, and MDMA-induced increases in sympathetic activity result in transient increases in heart rate and blood pressure and in pupil dilation.

In the brain, the monoamine neurotransmitters are synthesized and released by clusters of neurons (nuclei) in the brain stem: norepinephrine in the locus coeruleus; serotonin in the raphe nuclei; and dopamine in the ventral tegmentum and substantia nigra. The axons from these brainstem neuronal clusters extend, branch, and innervate large regions of the brain. Monoamine neurotransmitters thus have wide-ranging regulatory effects on global brain function, modulating attention, arousal, sleep, memory, and emotion.

Neurochemical actions at monoaminergic synapses propagate up to manifest global effects on brain electrodynamic activity, as measured, for example, by functional MRI. Ideas have been put forth as to how to interpret these global brain-activity changes and how they may underlie the well-documented behavioural effects of MDMA, but the limited research and the complexity of the system argues for caution in making strong claims as to global brain-action mechanisms (e.g. Carhart-Harris et al., 2015; Müller et al., 2021).

Animal studies beginning in the mid-1980s suggest that repeated high doses of MDMA are associated with reductions of serotonin and apparent oxidative damage to serotonergic axons, findings that have been called 'neurotoxic' (Baggott & Mendelson, 2001; Biezonski & Meyer, 2011). While this speaks to caution concerning frequent and/or high-dose use, there is no evidence for neurotoxic effects in humans for the dosages and frequencies of use employed in the clinical studies of MDMA-assisted therapy. Similarly, some studies have suggested that MDMA use may produce neuropsychological deficits. These studies frequently employ heavy users of illicit 'ecstasy' and are often poorly controlled with respect to other confounding factors (Mueller et al., 2016; Amaroso, 2019). Again, there is no evidence for neuropsychological impairment in the clinical studies of MDMA-assisted therapy (Clinical trials section, below).

MDMA also evokes release of oxytocin by oxytocinergic neurons in the hypothalamus, resulting in increased plasma levels of oxytocin and oxytocin-mediated neuroplastic effects in the nucleus accumbens (Thompson et al., 2007; Nardou et al., 2019). The effect of MDMA on oxytocin appears to be mediated by activation of serotonin receptors via serotonin released by MDMA's effect on serotonin transporters. As oxytocinergic activity is found to correlate with social interaction and reward, the effect of MDMA on oxytocin may be a contributor to MDMA's prosocial effects (Dumont et al., 2009). Oxytocin-mediated neuroplastic effects may also contribute to a reconfiguring of neural pathways in ways that stabilize emotional healing that may occur in a therapeutic context.

It is via all these effects (and doubtless more, not yet known) that MDMA presumably occasions increased arousal, wakefulness, and reduced psychological defensiveness—facilitating emotional exploration and greater ease in communication and connection with self and others. Something is happening in the brain and body that allows for a grounded examination of emotional pain, and the possibility of reconfiguring one's present connection with that pain—a corrective emotional experience of sorts.

The complexity of the brain limits our present capacity to do more than speculate on the details of mechanisms. Nonetheless, neurobiological images can be contributors to psychotherapeutic efficacy by highlighting that there are 'real' physical changes taking place in the brain and body associated with the MDMA-facilitated therapeutic experience. Of course, there are *always*, no matter what is happening, physical changes taking place in the brain and body. But it is also the case that whatever is happening in the presence of MDMA (and other psychedelic medicines as well) frequently has a lasting impact on behaviour—thereby contributing to the power and therapeutic utility of these medicines.

Clinical trials

Criminalization of MDMA in 1985 created regulatory and funding obstacles that seriously delayed progress in clinical research. At the same time, widespread 'recreational' use of the compound spurred governments around the world to fund preclinical research, which is a necessary step before clinical trials in humans are permitted. This government expenditure turned out to be important because the only clinical research program aimed towards regulatory approval of MDMA as a therapeutic drug has been funded entirely through a nonprofit group — the Multidisciplinary Association for Psychedelic Studies (MAPS)—testing the safety and efficacy of MDMA-assisted therapy for treating posttraumatic stress disorder (PTSD).

In these trials MDMA is administered during psychotherapy sessions to study its effect as an augmentation or catalyst to therapy (see also Chapter 2). In blinded, randomized fashion, MDMA or comparator (inactive placebo or low-dose MDMA) is taken only a few times (usually three) at monthly intervals during a seven-to-eight-hour therapy session with two therapists. These sessions are preceded by careful psychological and medical screening and by three preparatory therapy sessions. Each MDMA session is followed by three follow-up sessions aimed at helping participants integrate their experiences (Figure 4.2).

Between 2004 and 2016, six Phase 2 studies were completed, testing MDMA-assisted therapy as treatment for PTSD at five different sites in the United States, Canada, Switzerland, and Israel. Pooled results demonstrated a large effect size (Cohen's $d = 0.8$) for MDMA compared to improvement from the same therapy with placebo or low-dose comparator, which itself led to clinically and statistically significant improvements.

Side-effects were frequent, but well tolerated and self-limited. Most common were anxiety, dizziness, fatigue, headache, jaw clenching, nausea, and diminished appetite (Mithoefer et al., 2019). Blood pressure and pulse elevations were comparable to those seen with exercise, and never required medical intervention; participants had been screened to exclude underlying vascular disease.

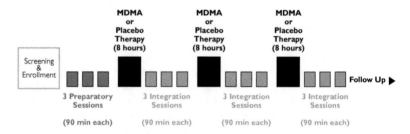

Figure 4.2 MDMA-assisted therapy: preparation sessions, MDMA sessions, integration sessions.

Because of concerns about possible adverse neuropsychologic effects raised by animal studies and studies in recreational users, neuropsychological testing was performed in two of the Phase 2 studies before and after two administrations of MDMA or placebo (Mithoefer et al., 2011; Ot'alora et al., 2018; Mithoefer et al., 2019). Testing used the Repeatable Battery for the Assessment of Neuropsychological Status (RBANS), which assesses function across five cognitive domains: immediate memory, delayed memory, visuospatial construction, language, and attention (Randolph et al., 1998). No effects were seen in any of these domains (Figure 4.3).

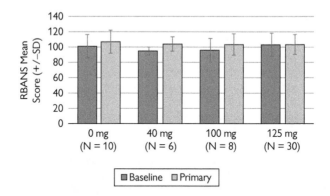

Figure 4.3 Neuropsychological testing using the RBANS before and after MDMA-assisted therapy for PTSD. Higher scores indicate improved performance. Baseline testing is prior to therapy. Primary testing is after two MDMA-assisted sessions. Testing done by Mithoefer et al. (2011) and Ot'alora et al. (2018). Data previously unpublished.

An additional secondary measure in Phase 2 trials was the NEO PI-R Personality Inventory (NEO), a well-validated inventory that characterizes human personality in terms of a five-factor model with six facets correlated within each specific trait. Results from a trial that enrolled military veterans and first responders indicated persistent significant increases in openness and decreases in neuroticism following MDMA-assisted treatment. Covariate analysis revealed that changes in openness but not neuroticism played a moderating role in the relationship between reduced PTSD symptoms and MDMA treatment. The authors (Wagner et al., 2017) argue:

> These preliminary findings suggest that the effect of MDMA-assisted psycho-therapy extends beyond specific PTSD symptomatology and fundamentally alters personality structure, resulting in long-term persisting personality change.

Based on the promising Phase 2 results, in 2017, the US Food and Drug Administration (FDA) granted 'breakthrough therapy' designation to MDMA-assisted therapy and gave approval to proceed with Phase 3 trials. Because of the strong subjective effects of MDMA, maintaining a double blind was one of the challenges in trial design (see also Chapter 11). In a series of Phase 2 studies, attempts had been made to improve the blinding by using various low doses of MDMA (25–40 mg) as a comparator. Maintenance of blinding was improved somewhat over that with inactive placebo; however, another confound was created—lower doses of MDMA increased anxiety and cut the benefit of the therapy in half. Subsequently, several Phase 1 trials by others have tested active comparators such as methamphetamine and methylphenidate. Both proved to have their own confounding effects on symptom measures (Bedi et al., 2010; Dolder et al., 2018). Based on this experience, Phase 3 trials were designed to compare therapy plus MDMA (dose range: 80 + 40 mg to 120 + 60 mg) to therapy plus inactive placebo in double-blind fashion. Effective blinding of raters was assured by using a centralized pool of remote raters. The FDA agreed to the adequacy of this trial design.

The first, pivotal, Phase 3 study was completed in 2020, across fifteen sites (Mitchell et al., 2021). The second, confirmatory, Phase 3 trial has been completed and results are pending at the time of this writing. Strongly significant results for the primary outcome measure (CAPS-5: Clinician-Administered PTSD Scale for DSM-5) in the pivotal trial are illustrated in Figure 4.4. There were no site differences in CAPS-5 response across sites.

Statistically significant improvements were also seen in the Sheehan Disability Scale and the Beck Depression Inventory. An additional finding that has not been demonstrated with other treatments was that participants with severe levels of adverse childhood experiences (ACE ≥ 4) and those with dissociative subtype on the CAPS responded as well as participants without those encumbrances. At baseline most participants had a history of developmental trauma (84.4%) or multiple trauma (87.85%). Mean baseline ACE score was 5.0. Nine participants

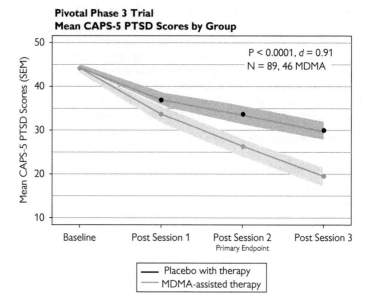

Figure 4.4 Mean CAPS-5 scores for MDMA-assisted therapy and placebo-assisted therapy for PTSD. Phase 3 clinical trials with eighty-nine participants, forty-six of whom received MDMA (Mitchell et al., 2021).

(21.1%) had a dissociative disorder subtype as assessed by the CAPS-5 (Mitchell et al., 2021).

In follow-up questionnaires and semistructured interviews during Phase 2 trials, participants had reported benefits that went beyond improvements in PTSD symptoms. Therefore, transdiagnostic secondary measures were incorporated into the Phase 3 trials, to track self-capacities associated with interpersonal functioning, emotional regulation, alexithymia, and self-compassion, using the Self-Compassion Scale (SCS), Toronto Alexithymia Scale (TAS-20), and Inventory of Altered Self-Capacities (IASC). MDMA-assisted therapy produced significant improvements not only in PTSD scores, but also in transdiagnostic variables that are likely to have a profound effect on overall functioning, specifically on affect regulation, negotiation of interpersonal conflicts, alexithymia, and self-compassion (van der Kolk et al., manuscript submitted). These results help to elucidate the psychological process accompanying improvements in PTSD symptoms. We hypothesize that they are also clues to the broader nature of a process of healing and growth that can be catalysed by MDMA-assisted therapy.

With completion of the confirmatory Phase 3 trial in October 2022, a new drug application to the FDA is likely to follow in 2023. In the UK and Europe, Phase 2 trials of MDMA-assisted therapy are being conducted in five countries and expected to start in two more in 2022. Meanwhile, several Phase 2 trials of MDMA-assisted therapy are underway at US Veterans Affairs (VA) medical centres.

MDMA-assisted therapy

The method of therapy used in the clinical trials discussed above is described in a treatment manual available at the sponsor's website (Mithoefer et al., 2017). The method is referred to as a relatively 'nondirective' or 'inner-directed' therapy and is based heavily on the approach developed by Stanislav Grof, one of the early psychedelic researchers prior to the criminalization of LSD (Grof, 2008). In MDMA trials, participants are encouraged to approach the MDMA-assisted sessions with as little agenda as possible regarding the course of their experience. The therapists aim to do the same. This is based on Grof's concept of an innate psychological healing capacity similar to the body's physical healing capacity. The hypothesis is that MDMA acts as a catalyst to accessing and expressing this ability. The role of the therapists is to remove obstacles and create favourable conditions for the healing process. Any direction they give or interaction they engage in is intended to support the participant's own unfolding process, not to direct it.

A few successful pilot studies have been published combining MDMA with other therapeutic approaches such as cognitive-behavioural conjoint therapy (CBCT) for couples (Monson et al., 2020), mindfulness-based therapy for social anxiety in autistic adults (Danforth et al., 2018), and treatment of alcohol use disorder employing aspects of motivational interviewing (MI) and cognitive-behavioural therapies (Sessa et al., 2021). Trials exploring MDMA for other indications, a diversity of populations, or as an adjunct to other established therapeutic approaches are under way or in development. Future studies will inform further innovations as the research progresses, and a range of choices for patients and therapists will likely result. Research thus far supports the value of an 'inner-directed' approach to MDMA-assisted sessions, even when they are combined with other more structured methods such as CBCT or MI during preparation and integration visits. This approach has produced large and durable improvements in PTSD symptoms in clinical trials. Whether substantially different approaches could yield comparable or even better results remains to be seen.

When an inner-directed approach is used in MDMA-assisted sessions, elements of other methods recognized to be therapeutic often arise spontaneously during MDMA sessions (Mithoefer, 2013). Both the degree to which and the order in which these elements arise vary with each individual and from one session to another. This variability offers the advantage of allowing each person's healing trajectory to unfold in its own unique way, with the therapists present to support rather than determine the trajectory. A few examples of themes regularly observed during MDMA-assisted therapy sessions are presented in Box 4.1.

As addressed in Chapter 11, limitations in maintaining a double blind in research with MDMA and other psychedelics naturally raise questions about the

---

Box 4.1 Examples of elements arising during MDMA-assisted therapy sessions

- Imaginal exposure, a central element in Prolonged Exposure Therapy, usually occurs in MDMA sessions without direction from the therapists, often with improved recall of events and the accompanying emotions. Participants typically report that processing trauma was still painful, but the MDMA effect helped them face it without feeling overwhelmed or having to emotionally numb to protect themselves.
- Participants often become aware of cognitive distortions and gain new perspectives without having to be directed to engage in cognitive-behavioural therapy.
- Regardless of the nature of the 'index trauma,' psychodynamic issues involving childhood and relationships are usually an important element of the therapeutic trajectory.
- The effects of MDMA often lead to increased trust, which allows for a corrective attachment experience.
- Effects may also include a sense of spiritual connection, awareness of the normal multiplicity of the psyche, powerful archetypal imagery, an increased awareness of somatic experience, and release of tensions in the body.

---

validity of the therapeutic results. There are several findings that provide reassurance about the validity:

1) Symptom reductions are usually maintained or even expanded at long-term follow-up of up to forty-two months.
2) Participants often describe a rich and coherent psychological process of the sort that would be expected to lead to improvement.
3) Symptom improvements are accompanied by personality changes of increased openness and decreased neuroticism.
4) There are significant reductions in disability as measured by the Sheehan Disability Scale.
5) There are significant improvements in secondary measures of self-capacities such as emotional regulation and self-compassion.

Valid assessment of the therapeutic potential of psychedelic-assisted treatments requires recognizing the importance of these findings, along with the results of quantitative measures in double-blind controlled trials.

Coda

These observations and models of therapy, as well as observations from neuroscience, shed light on some aspects of what is manifested in MDMA-assisted sessions during clinical trials. It is also clear that those aspects are only part of the picture. Extra-pharmacological factors play important roles; as Grof (2008, p. 49) puts it, these elements include:

> The role of the personality of the subject, his or her emotional condition and current life situation, the personality of the guide or therapist, the nature of the relationship between the subject and the guide, and an entire complex of additional factors usually referred to as set and setting.

Under the best circumstances, MDMA-assisted therapy may catalyse development of a capacity to revisit, without the drug, the state of conscious compassion and connection from which healing emerges. As Adamson puts it: 'It's almost as if the doorway to the heart-center, once opened, stays open, or can be opened very easily again, by choice' (2012, p. 171).

The phenomenology observed in therapeutic sessions with MDMA or other psychedelics points to the limits of our understanding about what additional factors related to psyche and world—who we are and how we conceive our relationship with what we consider as real—are central to psychological growth and healing. It invites our curiosity and our willingness to acknowledge that the complexity of what we observe goes beyond our current models (e.g. Grof, 1998). We are challenged to ponder what new perspectives and methods of exploration may be needed to approach understanding the depth and richness of the experiences research participants are reporting, and the levels of impact these experiences have on their lives.

REFERENCES

Adamson S (ed.) (2012) Through the gateway of the heart: accounts of experiences with MDMA and other empathogenic substances (2nd edition). Solarium Press. (Original edition, 1985; in the 2nd edition, it is revealed that Sophia Adamson is nom de plume for Ralph Metzner and Padma Catell.)

Amaroso T (2019) The spurious relationship between ecstasy use and neurocognitive deficits: a Bradford Hill review. International Journal of Drug Policy 64:47–53.

Baggott M, Mendelson J (2001) Does MDMA cause brain damage?, in J Holland, ed., Ecstasy: the complete guide. Park Street Press, 100–145.

Bedi G, Hyman D, de Wit H (2010) Is ecstasy an 'empathogen'? Effects of +/-3,4-methylenedioxymethamphetamine on prosocial feelings and identification of emotional states in others. Biological Psychiatry 68:1134–1140.

Biezonski DK, Meyer JS (2011) The nature of 3, 4-methylenedioxymethamphetamine (MDMA)-induced serotonergic dysfunction: evidence for and against the neurodegeneration hypothesis. Current Neuropharmacology 9:84–90.

Carhart-Harris RL, Murphy K, Leech R, et al. (2015) The effects of acutely administered 3,4-methylenedioxymethamphetamine on spontaneous brain function in healthy volunteers measured with arterial spin labeling and blood oxygen level–dependent resting state functional connectivity. Biological Psychiatry 78:554–562.

Danforth AL, Grob CS, Struble C, et al. (2018) Reduction in social anxiety after MDMA-assisted psychotherapy with autistic adults: a randomized, double-blind, placebo-controlled pilot study. Psychopharmacology 235:3137–3148.

Dolder PC, Muller F, Schmid Y, et al. (2018) Direct comparison of the acute subjective, emotional, autonomic, and endocrine effects of MDMA, methylphenidate, and modafinil in healthy subjects. Psychopharmacology 235:467–479.

Dumont GJH, Sweep FCGJ, van der Steen R, et al. (2009) Increased oxytocin concentrations and prosocial feelings in humans after ecstasy (3,4-methylenedioxymethamphetamine) administration. Social Neuroscience 4:359–366.

Freudenmann RW, Öxler F, Bernschneider-Reif S (2006) The origin of MDMA (ecstasy) revisited: the true story reconstructed from the original documents. Addiction 101:1241–1245.

Greer G, Tolbert R (1986) Subjective reports of the effects of MDMA in a clinical setting. Journal of Psychoactive Drugs 18:319–327.

Greer G, Tolbert R (1998) A method of conducting therapeutic sessions with MDMA. Journal of Psychoactive Drugs 30:371–379.

Grob CS (2000) Deconstructing ecstasy: the politics of MDMA research. Addiction Research 8:549–588.

Grof S (1998) Human nature and the nature of reality: conceptual challenges from consciousness research. Journal of Psychoactive Drugs 30:343–357.

Grof S (2008) LSD psychotherapy (4th edition). Multidisciplinary Association for Psychedelic Studies. (Original edition, 1980.)

Holland J (ed.) (2001) Ecstasy: the complete guide. Park Street Press.

Mitchell JM, Bogenschutz M, Lilienstein A, et al. (2021) MDMA-assisted therapy for severe PTSD: a randomized, double-blind, placebo-controlled phase 3 study. Nature Medicine 27:1025–1033.

Mithoefer M (2013) MDMA-assisted psychotherapy: how different is it from other psychotherapy? MAPS Bulletin 23:10–14.

Mithoefer MC, et al. (2017) A manual for MDMA-assisted psychotherapy in the treatment of posttraumatic stress disorder (version 8.1). Multidisciplinary Association for Psychedelic Studies (MAPS).

Mithoefer MC, Feduccia A, Jerome L, et al. (2019) MDMA-assisted psychotherapy for treatment of PTSD: study design and rationale for phase 3 trials based on pooled analysis of six phase 2 randomized controlled trials. Psychopharmacology 236:2735–2745.

Mithoefer MC, Wagner MT, Mithoefer AT, et al. (2011) The safety and efficacy of 3,4-methylenedioxymethamphetamine (MDMA)-assisted psychotherapy in subjects with chronic, treatment-resistant posttraumatic stress disorder: the first randomized controlled pilot study. Journal of Psychopharmacology 25:439–452.

Monson, CM, Wagner AC, Mithoefer AT, et al. (2020) MDMA-facilitated cognitive-behavioural conjoint therapy for posttraumatic stress disorder: an uncontrolled trial. European Journal of Psychotraumatology 11:1840123 doi.org/10.1080/20008198.2020.1840123.

Mueller F, Lenz C, Steiner, M, et al. (2016) Neuroimaging in moderate MDMA use: a systematic review. Neuroscience and Biobehavioral Reviews 62:21–34.

Müller F, Holze F, Dolder P, et al. (2021) MDMA-induced changes in within-network connectivity contradict the specificity of these alterations for the effects of serotonergic hallucinogens. Neuropsychopharmacology 46:545–553.

Nardou R, Lewis EM, Rothhaas R, et al. (2019) Oxytocin-dependent reopening of a social reward learning critical period with MDMA. Nature 569:116–120.

Nichols DE (1986) Differences between the mechanism of action of MDMA, MBDB, and the classic hallucinogens. Identification of a new therapeutic class: entactogens. Journal of Psychoactive Drugs 18:305–313.

Ot'alora GM, Grigsby J, Poulter B, et al. (2018) 3,4-Methylenedioxymethamphetamine-assisted psychotherapy for treatment of chronic posttraumatic stress disorder: a randomized phase 2 controlled trial. Journal of Psychopharmacology 32:1295–1307.

Passie T (2018) The early use of MDMA ('ecstasy') in psychotherapy (1977–1985). Drug Science, Policy and Law 4:1–19.

Passie T, Benzenhöfer U (2016) The history of MDMA as an underground drug in the United States, 1960–1979. Journal of Psychoactive Drugs 48:67–75.

Randolph C, Tierney MC, Mohr E, Chase TN (1998) The Repeatable Battery for the Assessment of Neuropsychological Status (RBANS): preliminary clinical validity. Journal of Clinical and Experimental Neuropsychology 20:310–319.

Rothman RB, Baumann MH, Dersch CM, et al. (2001) Amphetamine-type central nervous system stimulants release norepinephrine more potently than they release dopamine and serotonin. Synapse 39:32–41.

Rudnick G, Wall SC (1992) The molecular mechanism of 'ecstasy' [3,4-methylenedioxy-methamphetamine (MDMA)]: serotonin transporters are targets for MDMA-induced serotonin release. Proceedings of the National Academy of Sciences USA 89:1817–1821.

Sessa B, Higbed L, O'Brien S, et al. (2021) First study of safety and tolerability of 3,4-methylenedioxymethamphetamine-assisted psychotherapy in patients with alcohol use disorder. Journal of Psychopharmacology 35:375–383.

Shulgin AT, Nichols DE (1978) Characterization of three new psychotomimetics, in RC Stillman, RE Willette, eds., The psychopharmacology of hallucinogens. Pergamon Press, 74–83.

Shulgin A, Shulgin A (1991) PiHKAL (phenethylamines I have known and loved). Transform Press.

Stolaroff MJ (2004) The secret chief revealed. Multidisciplinary Association for Psychedelic Studies (MAPS). (Originally published as The Secret Chief in 1997, without identifying the secret chief as Leo Zeff.)

Thompson MR, Callaghan PD, Hunt GE, et al. (2007) A role for oxytocin and 5-HT1A receptors in the prosocial effects of 3,4 methylenedioxymethamphetamine ('ecstasy'). Neuroscience 146:509–514.

Wagner MT, Mithoefer MC, Mithoefer AT, et al. (2017) Therapeutic effect of increased openness: investigating mechanism of action in MDMA-assisted psychotherapy. Journal of Psychopharmacology 31: 967–974.

CHAPTER 5

Lysergic acid diethylamide: In search of the wonder drug

Mihai Avram, Felix Müller, and Stefan Borgwardt

KEY POINTS

* LSD is a potent perception-altering chemical.
* LSD has apparent anxiolytic, antidepressant, and antiaddictive effects.
* Modern studies indicate that LSD is safe to administer in a clinical setting.
* LSD decreases within-network but increases between-network connectivity.
* In healthy participants long-lasting positive effects are reported.
* No long-lasting negative reports have been reported by modern clinical studies.

> I believe that if people would learn to use LSD's vision-inducing capability more wisely, under suitable conditions, in medical practice and in conjunction with meditation, then in the future this problem child could become a wonder child.
>
> —*Albert Hofmann*

Introduction

Lysergic acid diethylamide (LSD) is probably one of the best-known perception-altering chemicals. It belongs to the so-called serotonergic hallucinogens or classic psychedelics and is classified as a semisynthetic ergoline (Nichols, 2016). It was synthesized by the Swiss chemist Albert Hofmann in 1938, but its psychoactive properties were discovered serendipitously only in 1943 (Fusar-Poli and Borgwardt, 2008). LSD has powerful psychoactive effects, including altered perceptions, audio-visual synaesthesia, derealization, and depersonalization, but it can also induce bliss and mystical experiences (Nichols, 2016; Holze et al., 2021b). Because of such dramatic effects, LSD was thought to be relevant for psychiatry and was introduced in the medical community in 1947 under the trade name 'Delysid' (see also Chapter 1).

Intriguingly, and perhaps unique to the medical field, LSD was intended not only as medication for patients but also for the attending mental healthcare professionals to 'gain an insight' into experiences of patients with mental disorders, especially psychosis (Nichols, 2016). Indeed, LSD's so-called psychotomimetic (i.e. psychosis-mimicking) effects spurred the first substance-induced model of psychosis (Geyer & Vollenweider, 2008). Paradoxically, LSD was also used as a therapeutic agent for distinct mental illnesses, including alcohol addiction, anxiety, depression, and psychosomatic disorders (Fuentes et al., 2019). Two psychotherapeutic approaches evolved: 1) 'psycholytic' (i.e. soul-loosening), which involved the application of small to moderate doses (30–200 µg), intended to intensify the psychotherapeutic process, and 2) 'psychedelic', which included the administration of high doses (300–800 µg) and aimed to induce so-called mystical peak experiences (Passie, 1997). Unfortunately, despite the strong research interest in LSD's effects and broad use in clinical settings, most early scientific investigations regarding its therapeutic efficacy do not hold up to today's standards (e.g. lack of standard dose, control groups, or blinding procedures).

In parallel with clinical interest, however, LSD became increasingly popular outside the medical community as a recreational drug. This uncontrolled use met with political pressure, which ultimately led to LSD's classification as an illegal substance (Schedule I of the *Controlled Substances Act*) and ban in the late 1960s. Severe restriction of using LSD and other psychedelics in research and medical practice followed (Fuentes et al., 2019).

Psychedelics, including LSD, have recently made a comeback, and their use in psychiatry appears to be gaining mainstream acceptance. The last decade has seen a revival of psychedelic research at several well-respected institutions worldwide (Tullis, 2021). Intriguingly, besides scientific interest, LSD is currently used in the treatment of specific, treatment-resistant patients in Switzerland and some other jurisdictions (so-called compassionate use).

Mechanism of action and clinical effects

The mechanism of action common to all classic psychedelics is mediated primarily via agonism at the 5-hydroxytryptamine 2A receptor (5-HT$_{2A}$) (Nichols, 2016). LSD is a partial agonist at the 5-HT$_{2A}$ receptor, but it also binds to other 5-HT (5-HT$_{1A}$, 5-HT$_{2C}$), dopaminergic D2 (less potently D1 and D3), and adrenergic α2 (less potently also α1) receptors (reviewed in Liechti (2017)). Notably, ketanserin—a 5-HT$_{2A}$ receptor antagonist—blocks LSD-induced subjective effects, demonstrating that 5-HT$_{2A}$ receptor activation mediates them (Holze et al., 2021b). The 5-HT$_{2A}$ receptor is expressed predominantly in visual and association cortices and less in sensorimotor cortices and subcortical areas (Nutt et al., 2020). The downstream effects of LSD are thought to be mediated by increased glutamatergic transmission, which is secondary to 5-HT$_{2A}$ receptor stimulation. These receptors are mainly localized on large pyramidal neurons in cortical layer V (but they can also be found on some GABAergic interneurons that regulate the pyramidal neurons) and enhance their excitability, which results in the dysregulation of ongoing brain activity (Nutt et al., 2020). Notably, these pyramidal neurons also project to subcortical areas such as the thalamus, possibly leading to aberrant thalamic gating (see The neural correlates of LSD below).

LSD, like all classic psychedelics (and some 'atypical' ones too, like the N-methyl-D-aspartate antagonist ketamine: see Chapter 9), appears to have (transient) clinical benefits (Nichols, 2016). For instance, LSD antidepressant effects have been suggested by early studies, and are supported by current evidence (Gasser et al., 2014). Anxiolytic effects have also been reported by early studies, and replicated by modern clinical studies investigating the effects of LSD on anxiety either with or without association to life-threatening illnesses (Gasser et al., 2014; Gasser et al., 2015; Holze et al., 2022b). Finally, LSD may have potent antiaddictive effects, as indicated by a meta-analysis of early studies investigating alcohol addiction (Krebs & Johansen, 2012).

The neural correlates of LSD

The first window into the brain on LSD was facilitated by studies using electroencephalography (EEG). Early EEG studies (1950–1960) demonstrated that LSD attenuated broadband spectral power in lower frequency bands (Fink, 1969). This result was replicated by modern EEG and magnetoencephalography (MEG) studies, which have also shown that reductions appear more evident in the alpha band (8–15 Hz) and that LSD enhances signal diversity and complexity (Carhart-Harris et al., 2016b; Schartner et al., 2017). Such changes appear to reflect a dysregulated spontaneous activity of cortical neurons, interpreted as an increase in the entropy of ongoing brain activity (Nutt et al., 2020).

Most studies investigating the effects of LSD on the brain used functional magnetic resonance imaging (fMRI), which enables functional brain mapping based on the blood oxygen level-dependent (BOLD) effect. Blood oxygenation changes link with local neuronal activity, which can either be experimentally manipulated (task-based fMRI) or investigated during intrinsic spontaneous activity (resting-state fMRI).

Task-based fMRI studies have shown that LSD decreases brain activation in areas related to emotion-processing (i.e. negative emotions), inhibitory control, self-processing, and social cognition. LSD reduces reactivity to fearful faces in the amygdala and medial prefrontal cortex (Mueller et al., 2017), which indicates a relevant therapeutic potential for LSD, as it contrasts with the bias towards processing negative stimuli seen in anxiety disorders and depression. Additionally, LSD impairs inhibitory performance on the Go/No-Go task by attenuating parahippocampal-prefrontal activation (Schmidt et al., 2018), which potentially facilitates visual phenomena. LSD also reduces task-evoked activation in the posterior cingulate cortex and angular gyrus, regions related to self-processing and social cognition (Preller et al., 2018b). This reduction contrasts with increased activity within the same regions reported for patients with depression, perhaps indicating another therapeutic potential for LSD.

Most fMRI studies, however, investigated the neural effects of LSD by examining changes in intrinsic brain activity (resting-state fMRI). Such changes can be measured by intrinsic functional connectivity (iFC) (i.e. statistical correlations between signal time-courses of different (sets of) brain regions). Studies have investigated LSD's effects on iFC in the whole brain, specific areas, or of intrinsic brain networks (IBNs)—reflecting functionally coupled brain regions. The main results of these studies can be summarized as follows: LSD (A) decreases within-network iFC (i.e. reduced network integrity), (B) increases between-network iFC (i.e. decreased network segregation), and (C) increases thalamocortical iFC with sensorimotor areas (Figure 5.1). Several studies reported decreased within-IBN iFC following LSD administration (Muller et al., 2018b). Intriguingly, one study found a correlation between reduced iFC in the so-called default-mode network (DMN) and the subjective effect of 'ego dissolution' (temporary loss of the sense of a self), which may have therapeutic value (Carhart-Harris et al., 2016b). However, this association warrants replication (Muller et al., 2018a). Notably, LSD-induced within-IBN reductions are not exclusive for the DMN, nor is the within DMN-iFC reduction specific for LSD, as other psychoactive substances have similar effects (Muller et al., 2021). Interestingly, increased iFC between typically segregated IBNs has also been related to 'ego dissolution' (Tagliazucchi et al., 2016). Furthermore, an increased global integration of distinct functional modules may also have therapeutic effects (Carhart-Harris & Friston, 2019). Finally, several studies identified LSD-induced iFC changes in thalamocortical iFC. Specifically, hyperconnectivity between the thalamus and sensorimotor areas was reported (for a review see Avram et al. (2021)). Such findings support a model positing that psychedelics elicit their effects by disrupting the thalamic gating of internal and external signals, resulting in the sensory flooding of the cortex, thereby giving rise to altered perceptions (i.e. hallucinations) (Vollenweider & Geyer, 2001). Intriguingly, the model also suggests that this disrupted thalamic gating mechanism underlies altered perceptions in psychotic disorders. Notably, 5-HT$_{2A}$ receptors appear to mediate

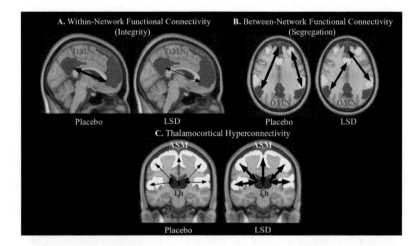

Figure 5.1 Putative neural mechanisms of LSD.
DMN - default mode network, SAL - salience network, Th - thalamus

some of the above-mentioned LSD-induced iFC changes (e.g. thalamocortical hyperconnectivity) (Preller et al., 2018a) but some neural effects may also be mediated by dopaminergic receptors (Preller et al., 2019; Avram et al., 2022).

Studies in healthy participants

Although some early attempts were made to establish the effects of LSD in healthy volunteers, the assessments were mainly conducted in comparison to (psychiatric) patients and are by today's standards scientifically suboptimal (Fuentes et al., 2019). Several modern, randomized, double-blinded, placebo-controlled studies have investigated the effects of LSD on healthy participants. Most clinical trials focused on establishing safety, effects of dosage, pharmacokinetics, pharmacodynamics, subjective and neural effects, and comparisons with other psychedelics (e.g. psilocybin) or psychoactive substances (3,4-Methylenedioxymethamphetamine (MDMA)) (Table 5.1).

Investigations of acute subjective effects following doses of 100–200 µg of LSD demonstrated a broad spectrum of hallucinogenic responses (Holze et al., 2019). The quantity and quality of these effects appear comparable to those elicited by other classic psychedelics such as psilocybin at certain dosages (e.g. 30 mg) (Holze et al., 2022a). Additional clinical studies are underway to compare between effects elicited with distinct psychedelics (NCT04227756).

Healthy volunteers perceive LSD's effects as largely pleasant, with some reports of acute negative effects (i.e. on a visual analogue scale) in 30%–50% of participants and a small number of overall disappointing/bad experiences (~8%) (Holze et al., 2021a). Acute subjective effects are closely related to changes in plasma levels of LSD over time, with maximal subjective effects being reached at 2.5 hours after administration, maximal plasma levels at 1.5 hours, and elimination half-life being around 3.5–4 hours (Holze et al., 2019). LSD pharmacokinetics are dose-proportional (i.e. for doses of 25, 50, 100, and 200 µg), and the duration of subjective effects increases from approximately seven to eleven hours depending on dosage (Holze et al., 2021b). Remarkably, participants could not accurately distinguish between 100 and 200 µg in this trial, as most LSD-induced reactions reached a ceiling effect at 100 µg. However, doses of 200 µg induced more anxiety, substantial experiences of 'ego dissolution', and 'anxious ego dissolution'. As positive long-term effects of psychedelics depend on the quality of the acute subjective effects (Schmid & Liechti, 2018), it is questionable whether higher doses are preferable for therapeutic purposes. For instance, LSD clinical applications in the 1950s and 1960s used very high doses—up to 800 µg (Fuentes et al., 2019). Regarding adverse events, doses of 50–200 µg appear comparable (Holze et al., 2021a). Although LSD significantly increases systolic and diastolic blood pressure and heart rate compared to placebo conditions, these alterations are moderate (Holze et al., 2021a). Overall, modern trials demonstrated that moderate to high doses of LSD can be administered safely under controlled conditions, with no long-lasting negative effects (e.g. psychotic symptoms) in healthy volunteers.

Table 5.1 Modern studies in healthy participants

Condition	CT Identifier	N	Status	Dose	Intervention	Location
Healthy	NCT04865653	20	Planed	100 μg/ 146 μg	LSD-base/LSD-tartrate/Placebo	University Hospital, Basel, Switzerland
Healthy	NCT04516902	24	Recruiting	100 μg/ 100 mg	LSD/MDMA/Placebo	
Healthy	NCT04227756	30	Recruiting	100 μg/ 20 mg/ 300–500 mg	LSD/Psilocybin/ Mescaline/Placebo	
Healthy	NCT04558294	24	Completed	100 μg/ 40 mg	LSD/Ketanserin/ Placebo	
Healthy	NCT03019822	28	Completed	100 μg/ 125 mg/ 40.03 mg	LSD/MDMA/ Amphetamine/Placebo	
Healthy	NCT01878942	16	Completed	200 μg	LSD/Placebo	
Healthy	NCT03321136	16	Completed	25 μg/ 50μg/ 100 μg/ 200 μg	LSD-25/LSD-50/LSD-100/LSD-200/Placebo	
Healthy	NCT03604744	28	Completed	100 μg/ 200 μg/ 15 mg/ 30 mg	LSD-100/LSD-200/Psilocybin-15/Psilocybin30	
Healthy	NCT02308969	24	Completed	100 μg	LSD/Placebo	

Population	NCT number	Enrollment	Status	Dose	Arms	Location
Healthy Ages: 55–75	NCT04421105	48	Completed	5 µg/ 10 µg/ 20 µg	LSD-5/LSD-10/LSD-20/Placebo	Not provided (Eleusis Therapeutics)
Healthy	NCT03790358	40	Unknown	6.5 µg/ 13 µg/ 26 µg	LSD-6.5/LSD-13/LSD-26/Placebo	University of Chicago, Chicago, USA
Healthy	NCT03934710	80	Completed	13 µg	LSD/Placebo	
Healthy	NCT02451072	25	Completed	100 µg/ 40 mg	LSD/Ketanserin/ Placebo	Psychiatric University Hospital, Zurich, Switzerland

Long-lasting effects of LSD in healthy participants have been examined in only two published studies, which found increases in openness and optimism two weeks after administration (Carhart-Harris et al., 2016a) and multiple, positive long-term effects (i.e. increased well-being, positive mood, and behavioural changes) up to twelve months after administration (Schmid & Liechti, 2018). Some positive changes were associated with the subjective effects 'mystical experiences' and 'blissful state', but also with overall drug effect (Schmid & Liechti, 2018). However, these outcomes need to be investigated in larger, placebo-controlled trials, as these studies were small ($n \leq 20$), and placebo control was missing in one of them (Schmid &d Liechti, 2018).

Several studies also investigated clinical efficacy of doses in the range 5–20 µg of LSD—so-called microdosing. 'Microdosing' is not clearly defined but refers to the practice of using repeated, small doses of a psychedelic to transiently improve mood, energy, or creativity in the absence of 'typical' hallucinogenic effects. Recent naturalistic studies (Ona & Bouso, 2020), along with some controlled trials (Bershad et al., 2019; Family et al., 2020; Hutten et al., 2020) have shown both nonspecific and specific hallucinogenic effects at doses of ≤ 10 µg LSD, with some negative effects at 20 µg. Other findings were inconclusive, with one study reporting enhanced attention and reduced information processing following microdosing, along with enhanced mood at doses ≤ 5 µg (Hutten et al., 2020), and two studies reporting no effects on the tested cognitive outcomes. Similarly, a recent study investigating the effects of four repeated low doses of LSD (i.e. 13 or 26 µg) in healthy volunteers reported no significant effects on mood or performance on cognitive tasks (de Wit et al., 2022).

Modern clinical trials with LSD

Current clinical trials investigating the potential therapeutic effects of LSD in clinical populations have mainly focused on patients with anxiety disorders (NCT03153579) and major depression (NCT03866252), but other potential therapeutic benefits are also being explored, for instance, for cluster headaches (NCT03781128) (Table 5.2). Completed clinical trials have shown that LSD-assisted psychotherapy is efficient in attenuating anxiety symptoms (assessed with the state-trait anxiety inventory) in patients with anxiety with or without association to life-threatening diseases (Gasser et al., 2014; Holze et al., 2022b), and that these effects are stable for up to one year (Gasser et al., 2015). Although promising, further evaluations are needed to clarify LSD's anxiolytic effects using alternative experimental designs (e.g. parallel versus crossover) and with better place control (active versus inactive placebo). LSD can be administered safely in patients with depression (Gasser et al., 2014), and preliminary results of a larger clinical trial investigating LSD's effects in depression (NCT03866252) will be available shortly. Notably, LSD's effects have also been evaluated in elderly healthy participants, to explore a possible role in the prevention and treatment of dementias such as Alzheimer's disease (Family et al., 2020).

Table 5.2 Modern studies in clinical populations

Condition	CT Identifier	N	Status	Dose	Intervention	Location
Cluster headache	NCT03781128	30	Recruiting	100 µg	LSD/Placebo	University Hospital, Basel, Switzerland
Major depression disorder	NCT03866252	60	Recruiting	100–200 µg/25 µg	LSD/Active placebo	
Anxiety disorders	NCT03153579	40	Active	200 µg	LSD/Placebo	
Illness-related anxiety	NCT00920387	12	Completed	200 µg/20 µg	LSD/Active placebo/ Psychotherapy	Private Practices of Peter Gasser MD Solothurn, Switzerland

l1 drug, which impedes research. Furthermore, LSD, more so than other psychedelics, has been at the receiving end of substantial stigmatization, which has damaged its image dramatically. In light of recent findings, legal authorities and others might feel inclined to revise their views of both the potential risk and potential value of this fascinating compound.

Future directions

The revived interest in psychedelics has not left LSD untouched. Modern clinical studies have established that LSD can be administered safely in a clinical setting, and they are currently exploring potential therapeutic effects in several clinical populations, ranging from anxiety disorders and depression to cluster headaches. However, many unknowns remain concerning LSD's clinical potential, as current knowledge relies on early studies and small sample sizes. While ongoing clinical studies may confirm anxiolytic and antidepressant effects, larger, placebo-controlled studies will be needed to establish its full therapeutic value. Crucially, some potential clinical effects of LSD have not yet been investigated systematically by modern studies, including likely anti-addictive effects (Fuentes et al., 2019). Future studies also need to determine which LSD effects are mainly pharmacological and which are driven by setting or parallel psychotherapeutic interventions. It also remains to be determined how long the clinical effects of LSD last after a single dose and if several doses may improve clinical outcomes. We acknowledge that these latter issues are not related to LSD specifically but rather to all psychedelics (see Chapter 11).

As detailed in Chapter 3, modern clinical studies have focused more on psilocybin than LSD, mostly because of the duration of LSD-induced subjective effects (8-12 hours, depending on the dose administered) (Holze et al., 2021b), which makes psilocybin more pragmatic. However, the apparent therapeutic effects of these substances need to be compared directly.

Finally, despite the increase in mainstream acceptance—including peaked interest of pharmaceutical companies and psychedelic stocks—LSD, akin to the other classic psychedelics, is a Schedule 1 drug, which impedes research. Furthermore, LSD, more so than other psychedelics, has been at the receiving end of substantial stigmatization, which has damaged its image dramatically. In light of recent findings, legal authorities and others may feel inclined to revise their views of both the potential risk and potential value of this fascinating compound.

REFERENCES

Avram M, Müller F, Rogg H, et al. (2022) Characterizing thalamocortical (dys)connectivity following d-amphetamine, LSD, and MDMA administration. Biological Psychiatry Cognitive Neuroscience and Neuroimaging 7(9):885–894. https://doi.org/10.1016/j.bpsc.2022.04.003.

Avram M, Rogg, H, Korda A, et al. (2021) Bridging the gap? Altered thalamocortical connectivity in psychotic and psychedelic states. Frontiers in Psychiatry 12:706017.

Bershad, AK, Schepers ST, Bremmer MP, et al. (2019) AcutesSubjective and behavioral effects of microdoses of lysergic acid diethylamide in healthy human volunteers. Biological Psychiatry 86:792–800.

Carhart-Harris RL, Friston KJ (2019) REBUS and the anarchic brain: toward a unified model of the brain action of psychedelics. Pharmacology Reviews 71:316–344.

Carhart-Harris RL, Kaelen M, Bolstridge M, et al. (2016a) The paradoxical psychological effects of lysergic acid diethylamide (LSD). Psychological Medicine 46:1379–1390.

Carhart-Harris RL, Muthukumaraswamy S, Roseman L, et al. (2016b) Neural correlates of the LSD experience revealed by multimodal neuroimaging. Proceedings of the National Academy of Sciences USA 113:4853–4858.

De Wit H, Molla HM, Berhsad, et al. (2022) Repeated low doses of LSD in healthy adults: a placebo-controlled, dose-response study. Addiction Biology 27(2):e13143.

Family N, Maillet EL, Williams LTJ, et al. (2020) Safety, tolerability, pharmacokinetics, and pharmacodynamics of low dose lysergic acid diethylamide (LSD) in healthy older volunteers. Psychopharmacology (Berl) 237:841–853.

Fink M (1969) EEG and human psychopharmacology. Annual Review of Pharmacology 9:241–258.

Fuentes JJ, Fonesca F, Elices M, et al. (2019) Therapeutic use of LSD in psychiatry: a systematic review of randomized-controlled clinical trials. Frontiers in Psychiatry 10:943.

Fusar-Poli P, Bogwardt S (2008) Albert Hofmann, the father of LSD (1906–2008). Neuropsychobiology 58:53–54.

Gasser P, Holstein D, Michel Y, et al. (2014) Safety and efficacy of lysergic acid diethylamide-assisted psychotherapy for anxiety associated with life-threatening diseases. Journal of Nervous and Mental Disease 202:513–520.

Gasser P, Kirchner K, Passie T (2015) LSD-assisted psychotherapy for anxiety associated with a life-threatening disease: a qualitative study of acute and sustained subjective effects. Journal of Psychopharmacology 29:57–68.

Geyer MA, Vollenweider FX (2008) Serotonin research: contributions to understanding psychoses. Trends in Pharmacological Sciences 29:445–453.

Holze F, Caluori TV, Vizeli P, Liechti ME (2022) Safety pharmacology of acute LSD administration in healthy subjects. Psychopharmacology (Berl) 239:1893–1905. doi.org/10.1007/s00213-021-05978-6.

Holze F, L Ley, F Muller, AM Becker, I Straumann, P Vizeli, ME Liechti (2022a) Direct comparison of the acute effects of lysergic acid diethylamide and psilocybin in a double-blind placebo-controlled study in healthy subjects Neuropsychopharmacology 47(6):1180–1187, 10.1038/s41386-022-01297-2.

Holze F, Peter Gasser, Felix Müller, Patrick C Dolder, Matthias E Liechti (2022b) Lysergic acid diethylamide—assisted therapy in patients with anxiety with and without a life-threatening illness: a randomized, double-blind, placebo-controlled phase II study, biological psychiatry, ISSN 0006-3223, https://doi.org/10.1016/j.biopsych.2022.08.025.

Holze F, Duthaler U, Vizeli P, et al. (2019) Pharmacokinetics and subjective effects of a novel oral LSD formulation in healthy subjects. British Journal of Clinical Pharmacology 85:1474–1483.

Holze F, Vizeli P, Ley L, et al. (2021b) Acute dose-dependent effects of lysergic acid diethylamide in a double-blind placebo-controlled study in healthy subjects. Neuropsychopharmacology 46:537–544.

Hutten N, Mason NL, Dolder PC, et al. (2020) Mood and cognition after administration of low LSD doses in healthy volunteers: a placebo controlled dose-effect finding study. European Neuropsychopharmacology 41:81–91.

Krebs TS, Johansen PO (2012) Lysergic acid diethylamide (LSD) for alcoholism: meta-analysis of randomized controlled trials. Journal of Psychopharmacology 26:994–1002.

Liechti ME (2017) Modern clinical research on LSD. Neuropsychopharmacology 42:2114–2127.

Muller F, Dolder PC, Schmidt A, et al. (2018a) Altered network hub connectivity after acute LSD administration. Neurolmage: Clinical 18:694–701.

Muller F, Holze F, Dolder P, et al. (2021) MDMA-induced changes in within-network connectivity contradict the specificity of these alterations for the effects of serotonergic hallucinogens. Neuropsychopharmacology 46:545–553.

Mueller F, Lenz C, Dolder PC, et al. (2017) Acute effects of LSD on amygdala activity during processing of fearful stimuli in healthy subjects. Translational Psychiatry 7:e1084.

Muller F, Liechti ME, Lang UE, Borgwardt S (2018b) Advances and challenges in neuroimaging studies on the effects of serotonergic hallucinogens: contributions of the resting brain. Progress in Brain Research 242:159–177.

Nichols DE (2016) Psychedelics. Pharmacological Reviews 68:264–355.

Nutt D, Erritzoe D, Carhart-Harris R (2020) Psychedelic psychiatry's brave new world. Cell 181:24–28.

Ona G, Bouso JC (2020) Potential safety, benefits, and influence of the placebo effect in microdosing psychedelic drugs: a systematic review. Neuroscience and Biobehavioural Reviews 119:194–203.

Passie T (1997) Psycholytic and psychedelic therapy research, 1931–1995: a complete international bibliography. Laurentius Publishers.

Preller KH, Burt JB, Ji JL, et al. (2018a) Changes in global and thalamic brain connectivity in LSD-induced altered states of consciousness are attributable to the 5-HT2A receptor. Elife 7:e25082.

Preller KH, Razi A, Zeidman P, et al. (2019) Effective connectivity changes in LSD-induced altered states of consciousness in humans. Proceedings of the National Academy of Sciences USA 116:2743–2748.

Preller KH, Schilbach L, Pokorny T, et al. (2018b) Role of the 5-HT2A receptor in self— and other-initiated social interaction in lysergic acid diethylamide-induced states: a pharmacological fMRI study. Journal of Neuroscience 38:3603–3611.

Schartner MM, Carhart-Harris RL, Barrett AB, et al. (2017) Increased spontaneous MEG signal diversity for psychoactive doses of ketamine, LSD and psilocybin. Science Reports 7:46421.

Schmid Y, Liechti ME (2018) Long-lasting subjective effects of LSD in normal subjects. Psychopharmacology (Berl) 235:535–545.

Schmidt A, Muller F, Lenz C, et al. (2018) Acute LSD effects on response inhibition neural networks. Psychological Medicine 48:1464–1473.

Studerus E, Kometer M, Hasler F, Vollenweider FZ (2011) Acute, subacute and long-term subjective effects of psilocybin in healthy humans: a pooled analysis of experimental studies. Journal of Psychopharmacology 25:1434–1452.

Tagliazucchi E, Roseman L, Kaelen M, et al. (2016) Increased global functional connectivity correlates with LSD-induced ego dissolution. Current Biology 26:1043–1050.

Tullis P (2021) How ecstasy and psilocybin are shaking up psychiatry. Nature 589:506–509.

Vollenweider FX, Geyer MA (2001) A systems model of altered consciousness: integrating natural and drug-induced psychoses. Brain Research Bulletin 56:495–507.

CHAPTER 6

Ayahuasca

Daniel Perkins, Simon G. D. Ruffell, and Jerome Sarris

KEY POINTS

* Ayahuasca is a traditional formulation consisting of the ayahuasca vine, which contains the harmala alkaloids, and usually one other DMT containing plant.
* The harmala alkaloids have MAO-inhibition activity, thereby increasing the bioavailability of DMT.
* The brew has a range of neurochemical effects which align with antidepressant, anxiolytic, and antiaddictive properties.
* Emerging epidemiological and clinical data exist for its efficacy in treating treatment-resistant depression, addiction, and trauma.

Introduction

The word 'ayahuasca' is from the Quechua language meaning 'vine of the souls' (McKenna et al., 1984) and is used by indigenous groups in South America to refer to a medicinal botanical decoction typically made from the *Banisteriopsis caapi* (ayahuasca) vine and the leaves of *Psychotria viridis* (chacruna) or *Diplopterys cabrerana* (chaliponga) (Ruffell et al., 2020). This psychoactive brew contains DMT (N, N-dimethyltryptamine) and harmala alkaloids, and has been used by indigenous cultures in the Amazon basin for healing, spiritual, and other purposes for at least hundreds of years (Shanon, 2002), with some evidence suggesting its use far predates this (Naranjo, 1986). Ayahuasca was also adopted as a religious sacrament by several Brazilian syncretic religions in the 1930s, and these have now expanded internationally to Europe, North America, and Australia (Lowell & Adams, 2017).

Recent decades have seen large numbers of international tourists visiting South American countries seeking ayahuasca's renowned therapeutic and spiritual or personal development effects (Peluso, 2016). At the same time there has been a rapid growth in ceremonies using ayahuasca or related preparations (involving alternative plant sources of DMT and harmala alkaloids) in underground indigenous-styled neoshamanic ceremonies taking place in countries across the world. This significant increase in popularity, and plethora of anecdotal evidence proclaiming the miraculous healing effects of the brew (Winkelman, 2005), has led many researchers to question whether DMT-harmaloid concoctions could indeed be safe and effective in treating some of the common mental health conditions we face today.

Clinical research overview

The use of ayahuasca in religious settings in Brazil has provided an unusual op-portunity to study effects of use among long-term drinkers. These studies have consistently identified individuals with prior drug and alcohol problems, including severe dependence, experiencing either complete remission or significant reduc-tions in use and apparent positive effects on mood and wellbeing (Barbosa et al., 2018). Furthermore, a systematic review of twenty-eight human ayahuasca studies reported that acute administration was well tolerated and that neither acute nor long-term use was associated with increased psychopathology or cog-nitive deficits (dos Santos et al., 2016).

Nonclinical and clinical studies, including a small number of double-blind random-ized controlled trials have reported evidence of antidepressant effects (dos Santos et al., 2016; Sarris et al., 2021b), antiaddictive effects (Perkins et al., 2021a; Nunes et al., 2016), and anxiolytic effects (dos Santos et al., 2016). Other research has reported therapeutic benefit in relation to PTSD (Nielson & Megler, 2014), eating disorders (Lafrance et al., 2017), borderline personality disorder (Dominguez-Clave et al., 2019), and Parkinson's disease (Serrano-Dueñas et al., 2001).

The one triple-blind placebo-controlled trial of ayahuasca to date was under-taken in people with treatment-resistant depression ($n = 28$), and it showed significant and rapid antidepressant effects after a single dose. The reduction in symtpoms of depression continued after dosing, and interestingly, a week later the experimental group showed a further reduction with a nonsignificant trend towards depression remission (Palhano-Fontes et al., 2019). Additional data from this study revealed that C-Reactive Protein (CRP) and Interleukin 6 (IL-6) (inflammatory biomarkers) were modulated by ayahuasca intake (assessed forty-eight hours post-ingestion) correlating with serum cortisol and a change in brain-derived neurotrophic factor (BDNF) levels (Galvão-Coelho et al., 2020). A significant reduction of CRP levels was observed across time in both patients and controls treated with ayahuasca (but not with placebo). The patients treated with ayahuasca showed a significant correlation (rho = 0.57) between reductions of CRP and lower depressive symptoms after administration (Galvão-Coelho et al., 2020). These data were also reflected in an eight-week social isolated con-text primate model, in which a single dose of ayahuasca reduced behavioural signs of depression and normalized cortisol levels compared to control (da Silva et al., 2019).

Broader psychological and wellbeing benefits have also been identified among healthy drinkers and those with mental health conditions. These include increased confidence, optimism, independence, and positive mood (Barbosa et al., 2009), as well as increased openness to therapeutic interventions (Winkelman, 2014). Some of these broader benefits can be summarized under the theme of 'Changed Worldview and New Orientation to Life', which encompasses fundamental life changes in terms of worldview, personal development, interests, and healing effects after consuming ayahuasca (Kjellgren et al., 2009). Ayahuasca-elicited changes have been documented in several mindfulness subscales, as well as emotional regulation, with one study finding improvements in 'acceptance' capabilities after a single ayahuasca session equivalent to an eight-week mindfulness training program (Soler et al., 2018).

A large observational survey of around 11,000 ayahuasca drinkers from more than fifty countries reported that ayahuasca consumption may beneficially affect alcohol and drug use, enhance mental health and wellbeing among healthy drinkers, and reduce affective symptoms among individuals with a prior diagnosis of depression or anxiety (Perkins et al., 2021b; Perkins et al., 2021c; Sarris et al., 2021a). A range of factors were associated with these positive outcomes including the strength of the acute subjective mystical experience, the number of ayahuasca sessions, and the number of personal psychological insights experienced. Adverse events reported were generally minor and transient, though some users did report emotional or psychological integration difficulties for which a small number sought assistance from a mental health professional, indicating that integrated psychological support may improve outcomes (Sarris et al., 2021a; Perkins et al., 2021b).

Psychopharmacology

Ayahuasca contains the classic psychedelic *N,N*-dimethyltryptamine (DMT), as well as several beta-carboline alkaloids that prevent enzymatic degradation in the gut (McKenna et al., 1984). Both DMT and the beta-carbolines found in ayahuasca have been linked to physiological and psychological markers of improved mental health (Aaghaz et al., 2021; Samoylenko et al., 2010; Barceloux, 2012).

DMT is a potent psychedelic known to produce radical shifts in consciousness, often characterized by profound visionary and emotional experiences (McKenna et al., 1984). Pharmacodynamic properties of DMT involve the modulation of serotonergic and dopaminergic signalling via serotonin-1A, -2A, and -2C receptor (5-HT1A, 5-HT2A, 5-HT2C) agonism, dopamine D2-receptor agonism, and sigma-1 agonism, with the psychedelic effects likely mediated via the 5-HT1A and 5-HT2A receptors (Fontanilla et al., 2009). Sigma-1 receptors are suggested to play a key role and be a potential target for addiction treatment, as well as being involved in the treatment of depression and anxiety, healing of traumatic memories, synaptic plasticity, and cell regeneration (Frecska et al., 2013; Sambo et al., 2018).

A further set of potential pathways associated with ayahuasca relates to the harmala alkaloids it contains—harmine, harmaline, and tetrahydroharmine. These compounds are MAO-A enzyme inhibitors, which serve to make DMT orally active, but also increase serotonin and norepinephrine levels, and have known antidepressant effects. Tetrahydroharmine is a weak SSRI itself, while harmine has been associated with increased levels of BDNF, the proliferation of human neural progenitor cells, and anti-depressive and anti-inflammatory effects (Dos Santos & Hallak, 2016; Liu et al., 2017). The psychotropic properties of harmala alkaloids (which belong to the group of β-carbolines derivatives) have been a matter of discussion since the early investigations of psychedelic drugs (Naranjo, 1967). β-carbolines have a diverse range of biological activities including an interaction with benzodiazepine receptors and 5-hydroxy serotonin receptors demonstrating sedative, anxiolytic, hypnotic, and anticonvulsant activities (Cao et al., 2007).

Together, the mechanisms of action of MAO-Is and DMT suggest a complex biochemical and psychological profile which may underlie therapeutic improvements purported from ayahuasca users (Ruffell et al., 2020).

Neurobiology

Ayahuasca has been found to activate brain regions such as the left amygdala and the parahippocampal gyrus. These regions have an important role in emotional processing and memory formation, while simultaneously modulating activity in higher cognitive regions—a combination thought to allow access to and processing of deep emotional material (Domínguez-Clavé et al., 2016). Key neurological processes proposed to be associated with the therapeutic effects include decreased connectivity in the default-mode network, reduced amygdala reactivity, decreased proinflammatory cytokines, and increased neurogenesis and neuroplasticity (Muttoni et al., 2019), as well as modulation of brain regions associated with interoception, affect, emotional processing, and volition (Riba et al., 2006). It has been suggested that ayahuasca temporarily modifies the ordinary flow of information within the brain by disrupting usual neural hierarchies (reducing high order cognitive control and facilitating bottom-up information flow), thus facilitating inner exploration and new perspectives on reality via the relaxing and revision of existing beliefs (McKenna & Riba, 2016). It has also been proposed that psychedelics may induce a unique window of adult neuroplasticity, described as 'critical period plasticity', like that of the adolescent neurodevelopment phase (Lepow et al., 2021). Neuroplastic effects are thought not only to be associated with psychological benefits, but potentially support the transdiagnostic application of a DMT-harmaloid based medicine (see Box 6.1).

Box 6.1 Summary of Ayahuasca's Mechanisms of Action

- Modulates serotonergic receptors (5-HT2A/C)
- Increases brain-derived neurotrophic factor (BDNF) in the brain
- Decreases in brain default-mode network activity and increased activity in brain areas such as the amygdala and parahippocampal gyrus
- Induces brain plasticity and neurogenesis
- Increases serotonin and norepinephrine and raises dopamine levels in the CNS

Psychotherapeutic elements

A range of potential psychotherapeutic mechanisms have been proposed for ayahuasca, listed below; combined, these changes in psychological skills are thought to contribute to improvements in various psychiatric conditions:

- Decentring: the ability to observe one's own thoughts and feelings in a detached, more objective manner (Domínguez-Clavé et al., 2019).
- Certain mindfulness capabilities: acceptance (nonjudgemental and nonreactive processing) and improved observation (Uthaug et al., 2018).
- Emotional regulation (Domínguez-Clavé et al., 2019).
- Experiential acceptance (González et al., 2020).

Ayahuasca has been linked to changes in a range of personality traits. Increases in agreeableness and openness, as well as decreases in neuroticism have been observed, with reductions in neuroticism correlating with the subjective intensity of the mystical experience (Weiss et al., 2021). Furthermore, ayahuasca-induced reductions in grief have been linked to increases in acceptance and the ability to psychologically decentre (Gonzalez et al., 2021). Cross-sectional reports of long-term ayahuasca users have found correlations between cortical thickness in the posterior cingulate cortex, frequency of ayahuasca use, and trait scores on self-transcendence—a personality measure of religiosity and spirituality (Bouso et al., 2015). Together, early work suggests ayahuasca may produce trait-level changes more rapidly than behavioural interventions targeting those specific traits.

A focus on the resolution of childhood trauma has been identified as a common motivation for people to participate in ayahuasca ceremonies. A likely rationale for this is that a core characteristic of the ayahuasca experience is a type of biographical review of important and defining life events (Wolff et al., 2019). A number of researchers have reported these processes to allow ayahuasca drinkers to connect with or uncover previously forgotten traumatic childhood events with a level of distance or perspective that facilitates reconceptualization and new understandings. Although this can be extremely challenging, it can lead to catharsis, healing, and new levels of empathy and acceptance for themselves and others (Fernández & Fábregas, 2014). Early data from the Global Ayahuasca Project also confirms these processes with around 50% of respondents reporting 'new understanding of childhood events or situations' as one of the insights or learnings they received during their ayahuasca experiences (Perkins & Sarris, 2021).

Clinical considerations

In general, psychedelic drugs are considered physiologically safe, although they can pose psychological dangers when factors such as set (the participants' mindset) and setting (aspects if the physical environment, including surroundings and the relationship with the therapist) are not appropriately considered (see Chapter 2). Accumulating evidence suggest this is also the case for ayahuasca, which has been found to be relatively safe and nontoxic (Guimarães et al., 2020). Data from randomized control studies consistently indicate that an individual's mental state prior to and during the acute phase, as well as the quality and intensity of the acute subjective experience itself, are key factors affecting clinical outcomes (Nunes et al., 2016).

Broadly speaking, it is expected that an ayahuasca-assisted therapy would be comprised of the same three components that are used in existing psychedelic-assisted-therapy approaches, as outlined in Chapter 2: 1) preparation for the dosing session, 2) support during the dosing session, and 3) debriefing and integration following administration. The dosing sessions take place in a specially prepared room, including a couch, artwork, and plants, with typical hospital room items removed or concealed. A specifically selected music playlist is advised to be prepared and used for all participants.

The psychological sessions occurring prior to a psychedelic medication session aim to develop therapeutic rapport with the participant, provide guidance about dealing with potential difficult experiences, foster personal goals for the session, gather information about the participant and their history, and provide psychoeducation regarding the acute experience, logistics, and therapeutic approach to be used and mutual expectations and boundaries. During the dosing session affirming nondirective support is provided, while the debriefing sessions assist in the psychological integration of the participant's experience. When the acute drug effects are strongest, verbal communication is minimized to facilitate the participant's inner experience. When these effects begin to dissipate, participants are invited to engage with the therapist and talk about their experience, personal insights, and emotions and evoked and to reflect on their journey. The approach aims to provide an attentive but nonintrusive empathetic presence. Emotional support and encouragement are also provided, inviting the participant to engage with difficult thoughts, sensations, or memories that arise.

Conclusions

As outlined above, there are encouraging data to support further controlled studies investigating the therapeutic use of ayahuasca to treat a range of mental health afflictions and addictions. However, important methodological issues must be noted in studies undertaken to date, including being primarily uncontrolled, small sample sizes, and difficulties with blinding. The medicalization of ayahuasca also raises questions regarding the formation of appropriate reciprocal relationships with communities who traditionally use this brew for medical and spiritual purposes (Wolff et al., 2019). Progression of the potential medical use of ayahuasca will require high-quality controlled studies incorporating a culturally sensitive approach to use used in a Western clinical context.

Acknowledgements

JS is supported by an NHMRC Clinical (Fellowship APP1125000).

Conflicts of interest

JS and DP are directors of a not-for-profit medicinal psychedelics research institute, which receives funding from commercial sources to facilitate research in this field. SR is employed at this not-for-profit medicinal psychedelics research institute.

REFERENCES

Aaghaz S, Sharma K, Jain R, et al. (2021) B-carbolines as potential anticancer agents. European Journal of Medicinal Chemistry 216:113321.

Barbosa PC, Cazorla IM, Giglio JS, et al. (2009) A six-month prospective evaluation of personality traits, psychiatric symptoms and quality of life in ayahuasca-naive subjects. Journal of Psychoactive Drugs 41:205–212.

Barbosa PCR, Tófoli LF, Bogenschutz MP, et al. (2018) Assessment of alcohol and tobacco use disorders among religious users of ayahuasca. Frontiers in Psychiatry 9;136.

Barceloux DG (2012) Ayahuasca, harmala alkaloids, and dimethyltryptamines, in Robert B Palmer, ed., Toxicology associates. John Wiley & Sons, 768–780.

Bouso JC, Palhano-Fontes F, Rodríguez-Fornells A, et al. (2015) Long-term use of psychedelic drugs is associated with differences in brain structure and personality in humans. European Neuropsychopharmacology 25:483–492.

Cao R, Peng W, Wang Z, et al. (2007) [beta]-carboline alkaloids: biochemical and pharmacological functions. Current Medicinal Chemistry 14:479–500.

da Silva FS, Silva EAS, Sousa GM, Jr., et al. (2019) Acute effects of ayahuasca in a juvenile non-human primate model of depression. Brazilian Journal of Psychiatry 41:280–288.

Dominguez-Clave E, Soler J, Elices M, et al. (2022) Ayahuasca may help to improve self-compassion and self-criticism capacities. Human Psychopharmacololology 37:e2807.

Domínguez-Clavé E, Soler J, Elices M, et al. (2016) Ayahuasca: pharmacology, neuroscience and therapeutic potential. Brain Research Bulletin 126:89–101.

Dominguez-Clave E, Soler J, Pascual JC, et al. (2019) Ayahuasca improves emotion dysregulation in a community sample and in individuals with borderline-like traits. Psychopharmacology 236:573–580.

Dos Santos RG, Hallak JEC (2017) Effects of the natural β-carboline alkaloid harmine, a main constituent of ayahuasca, in memory and in the hippocampus: a systematic literature review of preclinical studies. Journal of Psychoactive Drugs 49:1–10.

Dos Santos RG, Hallak JEC, Bouso JC, et al. (2016) The current state of research on ayahuasca: a systematic review of human studies assessing psychiatric symptoms, neuropsychological functioning, and neuroimaging. Journal of Psychopharmacology 30:1230–1247.

Fernández X, Fábregas JM (2014) Experience of treatment with ayahuasca for drug addiction in the Brazilian Amazon, in BC Labate, C Cavnar, eds., The therapeutic use of ayahuasca. Springer, 43–44.

Fontanilla D, Johannessen M, Hajipour AR, et al. (2009) The hallucinogen N,N-dimethyltryptamine (DMT) is an endogenous sigma-1 receptor regulator. Science **323**:934–937.

Frecska E, Szabo A, Winkelman MJ, et al. (2013) A possibly sigma-1 receptor mediated role of dimethyltryptamine in tissue protection, regeneration, and immunity. Journal of Neural Transmission (Vienna) **120**:1295–1303.

Galvão-Coelho NL, de Menezes Galvão AC, de Almeida RN, et al. (2020) Changes in inflammatory biomarkers are related to the antidepressant effects of ayahuasca. Journal of Psychopharmacology **34**:1125–1133.

González D, Cantillo J, Pérez I, et al. (2020) Therapeutic potential of ayahuasca in grief: a prospective, observational study. Psychopharmacology **237**:1171–1182.

Gonzalez D, Cantillo J, Perez I, et al. (2021) The Shipibo ceremonial use of ayahuasca to promote well-being: an observational study. Frontiers in Pharmacology **12**:1059.

Guimarães IC, Tófoli LF, Sussulini A (2020) Determination of the elemental composition of ayahuasca and assessments concerning consumer safety. Biological Trace Elements Research **119**:1179–1184.

Kjellgren A, Eriksson A, Norlander T (2009) Experiences of encounters with ayahuasca—'the vine of the soul'. Journal of Psychoactive Drugs **41**:309–315.

Lafrance A, Loizaga-Velder A, Fletcher J, et al. (2017) Nourishing the spirit: exploratory research on ayahuasca experiences along the continuum of recovery from eating disorders. Journal of Psychoactive Drugs **49**:427–435.

Lepow L, Morishita H, Yehuda R (2021) Critical period plasticity as a framework for psychedelic-assisted psychotherapy. Frontiers in Neuroscience **15**:1165.

Liu X, Li M, Tan S, et al. (2017) Harmine is an inflammatory inhibitor through the suppression of nf-κb signaling. Biochemical and Biophysical Research Communications **489**:332–338.

Lowell JT, Adams PC (2017) The routes of a plant: ayahuasca and the global networks of Santo Daime. Social & Cultural Geography **18**:137–157.

McKenna D, Riba J (2016) New world tryptamine hallucinogens and the neuroscience of ayahuasca. Behavioral Neurobiology of Psychedelic Drugs 1:283–311.

McKenna DJ, Towers GH, Abbott F (1984) Monoamine oxidase inhibitors in South American hallucinogenic plants: typtamine and beta-carboline constituents of ayahuasca. Journal of Ethnopharmacology **10**:195–223.

Muttoni S, Ardissino M, John C (2019) Classical psychedelics for the treatment of depression and anxiety: a systematic review. Journal of Affective Disorders **258**:11–24.

Naranjo C (1967) Ayahuasca, caapi, yage: psychotropic properties of the harmala alkaloids. Psychopharmacology Bulletin 4:16–17.

Naranjo P (1986) El ayahuasca en la arqueología ecuatoriana. América Indígena **46**:117–127.

Nielson J, Megler J (2014) Ayahuasca as a candidate therapy for PTSD, in BC Labate, C Cavnar, eds., The therapeutic use of ayahuasca. Springer, 41–58.

Nunes AA, Dos Santos RG, Osório FL, et al. (2016) Effects of ayahuasca and its alkaloids on drug dependence: a systematic literature review of quantitative studies in animals and humans. Journal of Psychoactive Drugs **48**:95–205.

Palhano-Fontes F, Barreto D, Onias H, et al. (2019) Rapid antidepressant effects of the psychedelic ayahuasca in treatment-resistant depression: a randomized placebo-controlled trial. Psychological Medicine **49**:655–663.

Peluso DM (2016) Global ayahuasca: an entrepreneurial ecosystem, in BC Labate, C Cavnar, AK Gearin, eds., The world ayahuasca diaspora: reinventions and controversies. Ashgate, 11–21.

Perkins D, Opaleye E, Simonova H, et al. (2021a) Associations between ayahuasca consumption in naturalistic settings and current alcohol and drug use: results of a large international cross-sectional survey. Drug and Alcohol Review **41**:265–274.

Perkins D, Sarris J (2021b) Ayahuasca and childhood trauma: potential therapeutic applications, in BC Labate, C Cavnar, eds., Ayahuasca healing & science. Springer, 105–106.

Perkins D, Schubert V, Simonová H, et al. (2021c) Influence of context and setting on the mental health and wellbeing outcomes of ayahuasca drinkers: results of a large international survey. Frontiers in Pharmacology **12**:623979.

Riba J, Romero S, Grasa E, et al. (2006) Increased frontal and paralimbic activation following ayahuasca, the pan-Amazonian inebriant. Psychopharmacology (Berlin) **186**:93–98.

Ruffell S, Netzband N, Bird C, et al. (2020) The pharmacological interaction of compounds in ayahuasca: a systematic review. Brazillian Journal of Psychiatry **42**:646–656.

Sambo DO, Lebowitz JJ, Khoshbouei H (2018) The sigma-1 receptor as a regulator of dopamine neurotransmission: a potential therapeutic target for methamphetamine addiction. Pharmacology and Therapeutics **186**:152–167.

Samoylenko V, Rahman MM, Tekwani BL, et al. (2010) Banisteriopsis caapi, a unique combination of MAO inhibitory and antioxidative constituents for the activities relevant to neurodegenerative disorders and Parkinson's disease. Journal of Ethnopharmacology **127**:357–367.

Sarris J, Perkins D, Cribb L, et al. (2021) Ayahuasca use and reported effects on depression and anxiety symptoms: an international cross-sectional study of 11,912 consumers. Journal of Affective Disorders Reports **4**:100098.

Serrano-Dueñas M, Cardozo-Pelaez F, Sanchez-Ramos J (2001) Effects of Banisteriopsis caapi extract on Parkinson's disease. Scientific Review of Alternative Medicine **5**:127–132.

Shanon B (2002) The antipodes of the mind: charting the phenomenology of the ayahuasca experience: Oxford University Press.

Soler J, Elices M, Dominguez-Clave E, et al. (2018) Four weekly ayahuasca sessions lead to increases in 'acceptance' capacities: a comparison study with a standard 8-week mindfulness training program. Frontiers in Pharmacology **9**:224.

Uthaug MV, van Oorsouw K, Kuypers KPC, et al. (2018) Sub-acute and long-term effects of ayahuasca on affect and cognitive thinking style and their association with ego dissolution. Psychopharmacology (Berlin) **235**:2979–2989.

Weiss B, Miller JD, Carter NT, et al. (2021) Examining changes in personality following shamanic ceremonial use of ayahuasca. Science Reports **11**:1–15.

Winkelman M (2005) Drug tourism or spiritual healing? Ayahuasca seekers in Amazonia. Journal of Psychoactive Drugs **37**:209–218.

CHAPTER 6

Winkelman M (2014) Therapeutic applications of ayahuasca and other sacred medicines, in BC Labate, C Cavnar, eds., The therapeutic use of ayahuasca. Springer, 1–21.

Wolff TJ, Ruffell S, Netzband N, et al. (2019) A phenomenology of subjectively relevant experiences induced by ayahuasca in upper Amazon vegetalismo tourism. Journal of Psychedelic Studies 3:295–307.

CHAPTER 6

CHAPTER 7

Ibogaine: Ibogaine therapy as a method of care treatment for opioid dependence

Deborah C. Mash

KEY POINTS

- Ibogaine is a psychoactive indole alkaloid found in the roots of the shrub *Tabernanthe iboga*.
- Ibogaine has been used widely in parts of Central Africa, notably amongst adherents to the Bwiti religion, as part of ceremonies marking 'rites of passage'.
- Open-label trials have shown efficacy for ibogaine in treating opioid dependence.
- Subjective reports underline benefit from the 'oneiric' visions associated with ibogaine, as well as a subsequent gaining of insight into the self-destructive behaviours associated with drug use and being more 'mindful' of the need to become sober or abstinent.
- Transient QTc prolongation has been observed with ibogaine and cardiac monitoring is required during dosing.
- Further safety and efficacy studies of ibogaine are required to allow full consideration of risk-benefit ratios.
- An ibogaine analogue is current being developed, with the hope of similar efficacy but better safety parameters.

Introduction

Ibogaine is a psychoactive indole alkaloid found in the roots of the equatorial African rain forest shrub *Tabernanthe iboga*. Ibogaine has a very long history of ethnobotanical use in small doses to combat fatigue, hunger, and thirst, and in higher doses, as a sacrament in Afro-Christian religious rituals (Goutarel et al., 1993). In the early 1960s, American and European self-help groups provided public testimonials that ibogaine alleviated drug craving and opioid withdrawal symptoms after single high-dose administration of the drug (Lotsof, 1995). Nonclinical studies in animal models of drug self-administration and withdrawal provided additional scientific support of these claims (Belgers et al., 2016). However, the evidence for putative therapeutic benefits of ibogaine are largely based on personal narratives and observations from open-label clinical studies. Today, thousands of people seek ibogaine treatment for substance abuse disorders in countries where the drug is unregulated. Online forums describe ibogaine use by for-profit clinics and lay-people to treat alcoholism and drug abuse, despite a lack of demonstrated efficacy and safety from human clinical trials.

Addiction is a behavioural pattern of escalating compulsive misuse, loss of behavioural self-control, and a high tendency to relapse. An integrated biopsychosocial approach is usually recommended to achieve recovery in substance-dependent patients. While ibogaine's effects on the brain are complex, the therapeutic benefits include rapid blockade of opioid withdrawal symptoms, reduced drug cravings and anxiety, and improvement in mood. Ibogaine may be a transformational pharmacotherapy for the treatment of substance abuse disorders because the drug's oneiric effects foster attentional focus on the problem, a readiness for personal change, and an improved quality of life following treatment. Despite these consistently reported benefits, there is a dark side to ibogaine which includes risk for adverse events when administered in unsafe settings. The outlook for ibogaine as a psychedelic medicine moving into the healthcare system for the treatment of opioid and other substance use disorders will depend on the benefit-risk analysis which guides regulatory decision-making for new drugs.

Historical overview

Ibogaine is one of twelve indole alkaloids isolated from the root bark of *Tabernanthe iboga* (Apocynaceae family). The forest-dwelling pygmy populations attribute the discovery of the plant to warthogs (Barabe, 1982). In parts of Africa where the plant grows, the bark of the root is chewed for various pharmacological or ritualistic purposes and ceremonial initiation practices of the Fang Bwiti religion in Central Africa, forming an integral part of their society (Pope, 1969; Fernandez, 1982). There are estimated to be approximately 2–3 million members of the Bwiti religion scattered throughout Gabon, Zaire, and the Cameroun, where ibogaine-containing 'iboga' or 'eboka' is taken in large doses as an initiation ritual, a powerful 'rebirth' ceremony that group members undergo before the commencement of their teenage years. The ingestion of iboga is supervised by the 'nganga', a senior Bwiti priest or priestess who has knowledge of iboga's effects on the mind and body. The purpose of this ritual is to allow the initiate to enter deeply into the subconscious mind with the intent of emerging reborn, a discovery that 'saves one from a confused and wandering state within the deep equatorial forest' (Fernandez & Fernandez, 2001).

A brief summary of the first one hundred years of discovery and development of ibogaine is shown in Table 7.1.

Discussion of the CNS and cardiovascular actions of ibogaine have appeared in the scientific literature since the early 1900s (Popik et al., 1995). In the 1950s, CIBA investigated ibogaine as an antihypertensive agent, but discontinued development since they were unconvinced of its commercial potential. The general interest in the Apocynaceae family of plants led scientists to pursue chemical,

Table 7.1 Historical summary of chemistry and pharmaceutical development of ibogaine

1889	Professor Henri in the 1889 session of the Linnaen Society in Paris offers the first botanical description of Tabernanthe iboga
1901	Ibogaine, the principal iboga alkaloid, is isolated from the roots of *Tabernanthe iboga* and reported independently by Dybovsky and Landrin and Lambert and Heckel
1930	Ibogaine is marketed in France under the tradename Lambarène until it is banned by the International Olympic Committee as a potential doping agent in 1966
1944	Delorme-Houda attributes to ibogaine the accepted formula C20H26N20
1957	Structure of ibogaine is definitively described by W.I. Taylor and colleagues from the CIBA Pharmaceuticals Research Laboratories in Summit, New Jersey
1966	Complete synthesis of ibogaine accomplished by G. Büchi
1970	United States Food and Drug Administration classifies ibogaine as a Schedule I substance
1985	Patent granted to Howard Lotsof for ibogaine as a rapid method for interrupting the narcotic addiction syndrome
1993	FDA grants academic investigators Sanchez-Ramos and Mash permission to conduct Phase 1 Pharmacokinetic and Safety Trial of Ibogaine

pharmacological, and behavioural studies of ibogaine (Pouchet & Chevalier, 1905; Lambert & Heckel, 1901; Phisalix, 1901). The French pharmacologists Lambert, Heckel, and Pouchet studied the pharmacology of ibogaine in the early part of the twentieth century (for review, Hoffer & Osmond, 1967). Ibogaine was marketed in France under the tradename Lambarene, as a mental and physical stimulant, until 1969 (Goutarel et al., 1993).

The putative antiaddictive properties of ibogaine were first described by Howard Lotsof (Alper et al., 2001; Mash et al., 2018), who reported that ibogaine administration of 6–9 mg/kg led to an active period of visualizations described as a 'waking dream state', followed by an intense phase of 'deep introspection'. Drug-dependent individuals imbibed ibogaine, report that their dream-like visions usually reflect on early childhood memories, traumas, or other significant life events. Some people recount that the experience gave them insights into their addictive and self-destructive behaviours. Opioid- and cocaine-dependent individuals report an alleviation or in some cases a complete cessation of drug 'craving' for extended periods, and some remain drug-free for several years thereafter following a single dose of the drug (Alper et al., 2001).

An informal addiction self-help network had provided ibogaine treatments from 1987 until 1993 to patients in Europe (Shepard, 1994). Based on his own experience and that of six of his friends, Lotsof formed a company and filed a series of use patents describing a method for treating narcotic, psychostimulant, nicotine, alcohol, and polydrug dependence with ibogaine (US Patents 4,499,096; 4,587,243; 4,857,523). In 1993 the Drug Abuse Advisory Panel of the US FDA granted an academic investigator-initiated Phase 1 Pharmacokinetic and Safety Trial in male subjects (IND 39,680; Mash et al., 2018). This clinical protocol was initially limited to include only ibogaine 'veterans' who had (previously) detoxed with the drug because of concerns of cerebellar toxicity demonstrated in rats treated with tremorgenic doses (O'Hearn, Zhang, & Molliver, 1995; Touchette, 1995). Subsequent studies in animals and a human neuropathology case report demonstrated species-specific and dose-related cerebellar effects that suggested a low risk for neurotoxicity in the dose range to be tested (Molinari et al., 1996; Mash, 1995). Based on these and other supportive data, the FDA-approved a revised protocol in 1995 to allow the Phase 1 studies to proceed in recently abstinent in cocaine-dependent male volunteers (Mash et al., 2018).

Psychopharmacology

Ibogaine is absorbed rapidly following oral administration and undergoes extensive first-pass metabolism to noribogaine (12-hydroxyibogamine) by cytochrome P450 2D6 (CYP2D6) in the gut wall and liver (Hearn et al., 1995; Obach et al., 1998: Mash et al., 1998; 2018) (Figure 7.1). Plasma protein binding is in the range of 65%–70% (Koenig et al., 2015; unpublished observations), and consistent with its lipophilic nature, ibogaine accumulates in fat (Hough et al., 1996). Maximum ibogaine concentrations in whole blood are estimated to be around 1,000 ng/mL, with maximum concentrations reached within approximately two hours. Noribogaine (12-hydroxyibogamine) is produced through metabolic demethylation soon after oral ibogaine administration (Mash et al., 1995; Mash et al., 2000). Ibogaine is cleared from the blood within 24 hours ($t1/2 = 4–6$ hours) depending on CYP2D6 genotype, while noribogaine is eliminated slowly over five to seven days following administration ($t1/2 = 24$ to 30 hours) (Glue et al., 2015; 2016; Mash et al., 2018).

Radioligand binding screens of the potencies of ibogaine at neurotransmitter receptor and transport sites in native members or cellular assays are shown in Table 7.2. Ibogaine inhibits transport of serotonin and dopamine with IC_{50} values in the low micromolar range (Mash et al., 1995c; Wells, Lopez & Tanaka, 1999; Baumann et al., 2001b; Jacobs et al., 2007). More recent mechanistic studies have demonstrated that ibogaine inhibits the serotonin transporter noncompetitively, in contrast to all other known inhibitors that are competitive with substrate (Bulling et al., 2012). In addition to targeted effects on serotonin reuptake and opioid receptors, ibogaine demonstrates pharmacological activity mediated in part by a noncompetitive inhibitory action on several nicotinic receptors, including the α3β4 subtype (Fryer & Lukas, 1999; Badio et al., 1997; Glick et al., 2000; Pace et al., 2004; Arias et al., 2010).

In animal models of addiction, the behavioural after-effects of ibogaine may be attributed to noribogaine, but these studies also show that the response

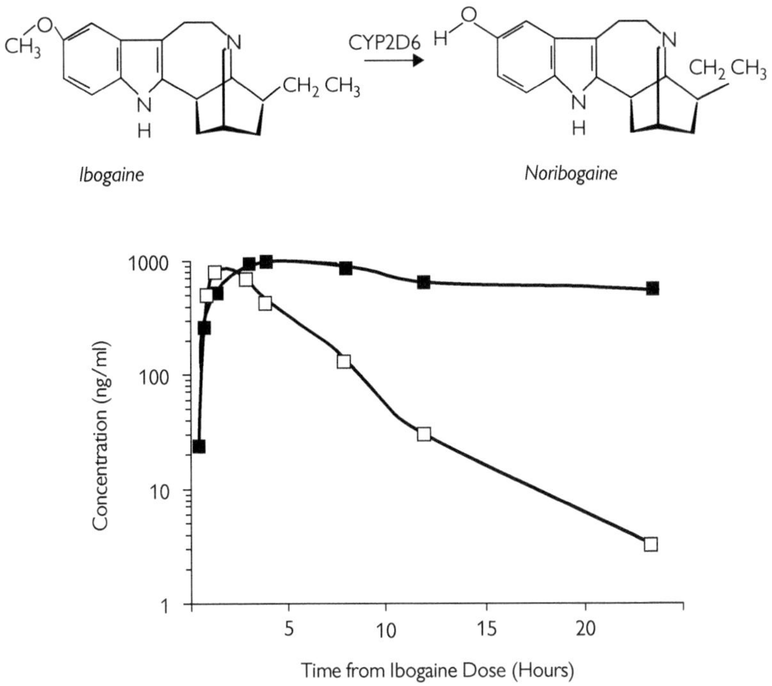

Figure 7.1 Ibogaine metabolism to noribogaine. The top panel illustrates that ibogaine undergoes O-demethylation to form 12-hydroxyibogamine (noribogaine) by the action of cytochrome

P4502D6 (CYP2D6). Ibogaine pharmacokinetics in a CYP2D6 extensive metabolizer (wt/wt) is shown in the bottom panel. Genetic polymorphisms in wildtype CYP2D6 influence the biotransformation of ibogaine in humans, resulting in complex pharmacokinetics (normal, intermediate, or poor (absent) metabolizers). The bottom panel illustrates that ibogaine (open square) is cleared from the blood while noribogaine (closed square) remains elevated postdose at the twenty-four-hour timepoint.

varies between these two drugs (Staley et al., 1996; Zubaran, 2000, Maillet et al., 2015). Ibogaine and noribogaine are not recognized as equivalent and cannot be fully substituted for each other even though their effects may partially overlap. Noribogaine binds to dopamine and serotonin transporters and kappa opioid receptors with equal or higher affinities compared to ibogaine (Staley et al., 1996). Noribogaine's affinity for the serotonin transporter is in the nanomolar range based on competition binding assays of the native protein in human brain membrane preparations (Staley et al., 1996). These observations suggest that the CNS activities of the long-acting metabolite in early abstinence may afford an added benefit by regulating low serotoninergic tone, which not only increases drug cravings, but worsens depression and anxiety. Hypoactivity of the serotonergic

Table 7.2 Binding-site affinities of ibogaine

Target	K_i; IC_{50}; Km* (µM)	Pharmacodynamics
Monoamines		
SERT ([^{3}H]5-HT reuptake; rat, human)	0.5–2.0	Serotonin reuptake blocker
SERT ([^{125}I]β-CIT (RTI-55) LLC-PK$_1$ cells) ([^{3}H]5-HT)	2.3; 0.17	Serotonin reuptake blocker Noncompetitive inhibitor of transport
Opioid receptors		
Mu (Naloxone binding, mouse forebrain; rat thalamus)	0.30–3.6	Agonist; partial agonist
Mu (DAMGO binding, rat; DAGO calf cortex)	1.0–11.0	Weak agonist/antagonist
Mu (DAMGO, HEK MOR cells)	19	Antagonist
Kappa (U69,593 binding, human)	2.0–4.0	Partial agonist
Delta (DPDPE, calf caudate)	>100	Inactive
Nicotinic ionotropic receptors		
Ganglionic (PC-12 cell line, human)	0.02	Inhibitor, noncompetitive
α3b4 nAChR (HEK cells, human)	0.22 1.0; 3.7	Inhibitor, noncompetitive
NMDA receptor		
MK-801 (rat cortex; rat forebrain)	1.0; 2.3; 3.2	Channel blocker
MK-801 (human caudate; frog spinal cord)	5.2; 9.8	Channel blocker
Voltage-dependent current (rat hippocampal cells)	3.2	Channel blocker

IC_{50} = half-maximal inhibitory concentration; K_i = inhibitory constant; nAChR = nicotinic acetylcholine receptors; SERT = serotonin transporter.

*The values of binding (K_i or IC_{50}) and functional assays (IC_{50}) and the pharmacological classifications are taken from several references and laboratory values (Baumann et al., 2001b; Mash et al., 1995b; Staley et al., 1996; Jacobs et al., 2007; Pearl et al., 1995; Codd, 1995; Toll et al., 1998; Antonio et al., 2013; Maillet et al., 2015; Badio, Padgett & Daly, 1997; Fryer & Lukas, 1999; Arias et al., 2010; Glick et al., 2002; Mash et al., 1995b; Chen et al., 1996; Popik, Layer & Skolnick, 1994; Popik and Skolnick, 1999).

system contributes to dysphoric mood states reported as part of the withdrawal syndrome (Koob & Volkow, 2010). Thus, the CNS mechanism of action for noribogaine may contribute to the lasting improvement in mood and diminished drug cravings following ibogaine detoxification.

The precise mechanism(s) underlying ibogaine's demonstrated rapid efficacy for opioid withdrawal management remains unclear. Ibogaine and noribogaine have been shown to modulate both the analgesic effects and physical tolerance to morphine (Bagal,1996; Bhargava et al., 1997) Although neither compound is a conventional mu opioid agonist or antagonist, binding affinities are in the low micromolar to high nanomolar range at mu and kappa opioid receptors (Pearl et al., 1995; Pablo et al., 1998, Antonio et al., 2013). Ibogaine and noribogaine fail to cause conditioned place preference of mu agonists or conditioned place aversion of kappa agonists or mu antagonists in animals (Parker et al., 1995; Skoubis et al., 2001; Maillet et al., 2015). In addition, neither morphine nor the full kappa agonist U50,488 substituted for the discriminative stimulus of noribogaine administration to rats (Helsley et al., 1998; Zubaran et al., 1999). More recent in vitro studies demonstrate that noribogaine is a G-protein biased kappa agonist and weak mu opioid antagonist with potencies that match physiologically relevant brain concentrations following administration of ibogaine in animal models (Maillet et al., 2015). Thus, noribogaine's atypical properties on the kappa opioid system and to a lesser extent on the mu opioid system should be considered as its potential mechanism of action of the metabolite acting on endogenous opioids (Maillet et al., 2015; Mash et al., 2016).

In vitro assays demonstrate that ibogaine is an NMDA receptor antagonist that binds to the glutamate channel (Mash, Staley, Pablo, et al., 1995; Staley et al., 1996; Skolnick, 2001). Pharmacologically relevant concentrations of ibogaine produce a voltage-dependent block of NMDA receptors. Moreover, ibogaine substitutes as a discriminative stimulus (ED50, 64.9 mg/kg) in mice trained to discriminate the NMDA antagonist, dizocilpine from saline (Skolnick 2001). Since noribogaine binds with lower potency as compared to ibogaine, it is unlikely that the NMDA receptor antagonism is additive to ibogaine (Mash et al., 1995b). This observation suggests that the 'oneiric' effects of ibogaine administration may be similar to the dissociative anaesthetic ketamine.

Rodent models suggest that ibogaine administration causes EEG gamma band alterations and REM-like traits that compare to natural REM sleep (Gonzalez et al., 2021). This provides novel biological evidence for a possible association between ibogaine's psychedelic state and REM sleep. If ibogaine's 'oneiric' waking dream state results from the engagement of neural processing associated with sleep and dreams, this activation state may be relevant for understanding how the drug 'resets' the brain reward circuit, including the ventral tegmental area and the nucleus accumbens (NAcc), which are known to be activated during sleep (Solms, 2000; Perogamvros & Schwartz, 2012). Perogamvrosa and Schwartz (2012) presented their 'Reward Activation Model' of sleep and dreams to integrate neurophysiological, neuroimaging, and clinical findings that point to significant activation of the mesolimbic dopaminergic (ML-DA) reward system during both NREM (N2 in humans, SWS in rats) and REM sleep. The authors suggest that dysregulation of such motivational/emotional processes attributable to sleep disturbances (e.g. insomnia, sleep deprivation) would predispose to reward-related disorders, including increased risk-taking and compulsive behaviours in vulnerable populations who are addicted.

Of note, Morpheus—the Greek god of sleep and dreams—gave his name to morphine. Opium and synthetic opioid drugs are sedating and produce a dream-like euphoria, which over time lead to markedly disrupted sleep architecture and insomnia following withdrawal from use (Valentino & Volkow, 2020). Sleep disorders are risk factors for substance abuse, and their severity correlates with alcohol, cocaine, and heroin use and relapse (Dolson et al., 2017). Further investigation into ibogaine's neurophysiological effects on REM and NREM sleep states in humans may be relevant for understanding why its 'oneiric' effects may benefit drug-dependent individuals. Since the endogenous opioid system plays a role in regulating sleep, multivariate EEG studies of drug-induced cortical activity may advance a better mechanistic description of ibogaine as a purported addiction 'interrupter'.

Understanding how ibogaine produces a 'reset' of addiction circuitry in the brain is an area of active investigation. Ibogaine and its metabolite are 'psychoplastogens' that have effects on dopamine circuitry through activation of glial-derived growth factor and other second messenger signalling pathways (Olson et al., 2018; Carnicella et al., 2010). Like other classic psychedelics, NMDA receptor blockade and 5-HT circuit mechanisms may explain the drug's dose-related 'oneiric' effects in humans, whilst noribogaine may mediate some of the beneficial after-effects of ibogaine administration through dynorphin-kappa and serotonergic mechanisms (Mash et al., 2016; Maillet et al., 2015). Reward hyposensitivity and anhedonia are associated with substance use disorders, and their severity is especially prominent in drug use disorders associated with comorbid depression (Destoop et al., 2019). The polypharmacy actions of ibogaine and its active metabolite may lessen withdrawal related anhedonia and improve other dysregulated reward-related circuits, with implications for being able to target multilevel aspects of substance abuse disorders.

Clinical observations

Patients physically dependent on opioids have described significant attenuation of withdrawal symptoms within several hours of ingesting ibogaine, with subsequently sustained resolution of the opioid withdrawal syndrome (Alper et al., 1999; Mash et al., 2001; Mash et al., 2018). Self-treating heroin abusers made the original discovery in the 1960s that a single dose of ibogaine essentially eliminates opioid withdrawal symptoms (Alper et al., 1999). Out of thirty-three human subjects treated with 6–29 mg/kg ibogaine (average 19 mg/kg), twenty-five reported amelioration of opioid withdrawal symptoms and no further desire to take heroin in the days following treatment. Results from a later, small case series of opioid-dependent patients seeking detoxification using lower oral doses of ibogaine (10–12 mg/kg) demonstrated similar results (Mash et al., 1998). Open-label studies of patients treated in Mexico (Brown & Alper, 2018; Davis et al., 2017), New Zealand (Noller et al., 2018), and St. Kitts, West Indies, (Mash et al., 2018) have demonstrated similar beneficial effects.

Academic investigators have advanced open-label studies of ibogaine's safety and effectiveness for detoxifying from opioids, cocaine, and other substances (Table 7.3). Brown and Alper (2018) reported results from thirty individuals (twenty-five men) meeting DSM-IV criteria for opioid dependence, treated with

Table 7.3 Human clinical experience

Ibogaine Clinical Study	Title	Study Design and Dose Range	(n)	Clinical Endpoints	Reference
University of Miami General Clinical Research Center	Ibogaine HCl IND39,680 Phase 1 Pharmacokinetic / Pharmacodynamic Clinical Trial	Open-label Phase 1 ascending ibogaine HCl (Omnichem, Belgium) dose (1 to 8 mg/kg po) ibogaine veterans (N=3; 1 mg/kg) and abstinent cocaine-dependent patients (N=6; 2 mg/kg)	9	Pharmacokinetics and Safety	Mash, unpublished
Mexico private clinics	Ibogaine in Patients seeking Opioid Detoxification under Medical Monitor	Open-label observational study in DSM-IV opioid-dependent patients, 12-month follow-up assessments, mean dose ibogaine HCl 1,540 ± 920 mg; extract of T. Iboga root bark (mean dose 1610 ± 1650 mg)	30	SOWS, ASI Composite and Drug Use Scores	Brown & Alper, 2018
New Zealand Physician administered, Practice Setting, Addiction Counselor referral	Ibogaine Treatment Providers Outcomes Study	12-month open-label follow-up observational study, ibogaine HCl 25–55 mg/kg (mean 31.4, SD 7.6); staggered dosing regimen, patient based; EU drug manufacturer and Canadian company, Phytostan Enterprises, Inc. Remogen drug product	20	SOWS, Addiction Severity Index-Lite (ASI-Lite), Beck's Depression Inventory (BDI)	Noller et al., 2018

(continued)

Table 7.3 Continued					
Ibogaine Clinical Study	**Title**	**Study Design and Dose Range**	**(n)**	**Clinical Endpoints**	**Reference**
Mexico Crossroads Treatment Centre Physician administered	Ibogaine-Assisted Detoxification Program for Individuals with Opioid Use Disorders	IRB-approved open-label online anonymous, web-based survey regarding patient experiences with, and effectiveness of, ibogaine treatment; Canadian company, Phytostan Enterprises, Inc. Remogen Product	88	Questionnaires, Subjective Effectiveness; opioid use before and after treatment; Depression, Anxiety, and Stress Scale; Satisfaction With Life Survey	Davis et al., 2018
St Kitts, West Indies, Ibogaine HVI Clinic Physician administered	Ibogaine-Assisted Detoxification of Opioid and Cocaine Dependent Patients; Other Substance Use Disorders	Open-label safety, pharmacokinetics and pharmacodynamics of ibogaine in patients with DSM-IV opioid or cocaine dependence (N= 191). *Polydrug, alcohol and amphetamine dependence (N=86) ibogaine HCl (99.8%) (partial weight-based dose, 6 to 14 mg/ kg po) Postdose and 1-month follow-up assessments; IRB-approved retrospective chart reviews	277	Adverse Events, CYP2D6 Genotyping, Pharmacokinetics, OWS, BDI, POMS, SCL-90, ASI, Heroin Craving Questionnaire-Now (HCQN), Cocaine Craving CCQN and Minnesota Cocaine Craving Scales, Elicitation Narrative with content coding	Mash et al., 2018 *Unpublished

a mean total dose of 1,540 ± 920 mg ibogaine HCl. There was a significant decrease in Subjective Opioid Withdrawal Scale (SOWS: the primary outcome) scores from pretreatment baseline (N = 27; t = 7.07, df = 26, p < .001) to 76.5 ± 30 hours after drug administration. The Addiction Severity Index (ASI) Composite Drug Use and Legal and Family/Social Status scores also showed improvement relative to pretreatment baseline at all posttreatment time points (p < .001). Drug Use scores from the ASI had maximal improvement at one month and to a variable extent over the subsequent twelve months.

The largest open-label investigation of self-referred patients seeking treatment with ibogaine for opioid (N = 102) or cocaine (N = 89) detoxification was conducted in St. Kitts (Mash et al., 2018). In this twelve-day inpatient study, opioid- and cocaine-dependent men (n = 144) and women (n = 47) all met DSM-IV criteria for opioid or cocaine dependence and had positive urine screens at program entry. The average age of the opioid-dependent patients was 35.8 ± 9.9 years, with lifetime use of 11.2 ± 8.6 years. Results demonstrated that single oral doses of ibogaine (partial weight-based dosage; 800–1,000 mg total) were associated with significant reductions in withdrawal symptoms and drug cravings, which persisted over the residential treatment period. Withdrawal symptoms according to the physician-rated OWS (score range of 0–13) ranges from 3 to 13, predose (taken twelve hours after the last opioid dose). Objective signs of opioid withdrawal at twenty-four hours following ibogaine administration were mild, and breakthrough symptoms were not observed at later times. Insomnia was a common complaint among opioid-dependent patients, which improved within several days following ibogaine treatment. All participants completed the planned duration of inpatient stay, and none returned to opioid use during the inpatient treatment.

Significantly decreased cravings for opioids and cocaine were observed at seven and at thirty days after ibogaine treatment using the Heroin (HCQ-29) and Cocaine (CCQ-45) Craving Questionnaires (Mash et al., 2018). There were rapid and sustained improvements in mood after ibogaine administration from baseline to postdose and at one-month follow-up (p ≤ 0.01).

In terms of subjective effects, participants described active 'dream-like' visions, beginning approximately thirty to forty-five minutes after ingestion (Mash et al., 2018). Sensory and perceptual changes included lucid imagery, changes in the quality and rate of thinking, and heightened sensitivity to sound. Most of these effects lasted between four and eight hours, after which there was an abrupt change to a period of deep introspection. According to a semistructured elicitation narrative, over 90% of participants reported deriving benefit from the 'oneiric' visions; a similar percentage endorsed ibogaine as beneficial treating drug dependence. Some patients described that they had gained insight into their self-destructive behaviours and that they were 'mindful' of the need to become sober or abstinent now (N = 50%). These observations suggest that ibogaine treatment may promote better outcomes for some patients because the psychedelic effects of the drug activates reasoning and decision-making following detoxification.

Noller et al. (2018) conducted a twelve-month follow-up observational case series ($n = 14$, 7 men; mean age $38 + 4.8$ y) of people seeking treatment for opioid dependence and who had used methadone ($n = 10$), codeine ($n = 3$), or excessive amounts of poppy seed tea ($n = 1$) in the thirty days prior to treatment. Participants received high doses of ibogaine (25–55 mg/kg; mean 30.4 mg/kg) with concomitant benzodiazepine and sleep aids if needed. The ASI (the primary outcome) showed significant decreases over time ($p = 0.002$), with a >80% decrease in overall drug use score from baseline to twelve-month follow-up ($p = 0.004$). The SOWS revealed a significant reduction in withdrawal symptoms from the predose timepoint following discontinuation of opioids up to the twenty-four-hour postdose assessment ($p = 0.015$). Depression improved ($p < 0.001$), apart from at the immediate postdose timepoint. Random drug screens yielded positive results for one patient each at three and six months and for two of the fourteen participants at twelve months.

In a separate study, Davis et al. (2018) collected subjective data (anonymous online collection) from eighty-eight individuals who had received ibogaine ($15 + 5$ mg/kg) as part of an opioid treatment program. Most participants (72%) had been using heroin or prescription opioids for four or more years, and some much longer (21% at least ten years). A total of 80% of the respondents endorsed that ibogaine eliminated or significantly reduced OWS, whilst 50% reported that ibogaine reduced opioid craving (25% reporting a reduction in craving lasting at least three months). A third of participants reported never using opioids again following ibogaine treatment, and half of abstainers had maintained abstinence for one year and one-third for two years posttreatment. The authors acknowledged several methodological limitations including that those participants who were unable to be contacted or who declined to participate most likely had different outcomes following treatment.

Further data on ibogaine in opioid withdrawal include an inpatient study from Panama in which physicians reported no objective opioid withdrawal symptoms, cravings, or drug-seeking in any of the patients at twenty-four hours post dose (Luciano, 1998). In a Mexican study, Camlin et al. (2018) performed face-to-face interviews with ten patients treated with ibogaine for detoxification; all reported complete alleviation and lasting attenuation of withdrawal symptoms and minimal to no drug cravings, but unfortunately there was no long-term follow-up.

Concerns for safety

Open-label investigations suggest a favourable benefit-risk ratio for ibogaine when administered under qualified medical supervision for opioid withdrawal (Mash et al., 2018; Luz & Mash, 2021). However, there are a total of thirty-three suspected drug-related deaths cited in the literature (for review, Corkery, 2018; Luz & Mash, 2021). Most of these fatalities occurred in unsafe settings in the absence of competent medical oversight. Causality assessments suggest contributing factors include CYP2D6-mediated drug-drug interactions, polydrug abuse, alcohol withdrawal, concurrent methadone use, undiagnosed cardiovascular disease, electrolyte (K^+ and Mg^{++}) abnormalities, impure drug product, or toxic doses of ibogaine (Luz & Mash, 2021). Opioid withdrawal itself can lead to severe fluid loss and electrolyte abnormalities that can contribute to cardiovascular instability and death (Darke et al., 2017).

Ibogaine has been shown to inhibit cardiac voltage-gated ion channels, including hERG potassium, Nav1.5 sodium, and Cav1.2 calcium channels (Koenig et a., 2014; 2015). Ibogaine's potency at hERG channels ranges from 0.8 to 3.9 µM. Blockade of the hERG channel is known to cause QT/QTc prolongation. However, these biomarkers are not the direct risks of Torsade des Points (TdP) based on the acknowledged low specificity (Vicente et al., 2019).

A recent open-label study examined ibogaine safety in fourteen patients with opioid use disorder who were on opioid maintenance treatment but had failed to reach abstinence (Knuijver et al., 2022). After conversion to morphine-sulphate, a single dose of ibogaine HCl (10 mg/kg) was administered and patients were monitored for at least twenty-four hours, using ECGs, blood pressure, and heart rate; they were also assessed for cerebellar ataxia (SARA), and the delirium observation scale was administered. The authors interpreted their results as indicating that ibogaine is an unsafe drug due to QTc prolongation and potential severe ataxia. However, the observed ataxia was transient and is expected at this dose range; SARA scores returned to baseline after the ibogaine was cleared, in keeping with pharmacokinetic parameters reported elsewhere (Mash et al., 2001; Mash et al., 2018). In practice, patients are required to remain in a supine position during the active 'oneiric' phase, which lasts between four and eight hours depending on CYP2D6 metabolizer status (Mash et al., 2018).

The authors reported concerning increases in QTc intervals. In seven of the fourteen patients, QTc prolongation was above 500 msec. Questions regarding the study design underscore some potential methodological issues for estimating the magnitude of the QTc interval prolongation. During the active 'oneiric' phase, heart rate fluctuations may contribute to the high intraindividual variability of QTc intervals (Knuijver et al., 2022; Supporting information, Figure S5). Therefore, subject-specific heart rate corrections based on full profiles derived from placebo baseline recordings with wide QT/RR distribution are needed to determine precisely the proarrhythmia risk of this biomarker (Malik et al., 2018). Also, opioid withdrawal alters sympathetic/parasympathetic outflow. Ibogaine may have centrally mediated effects which alter autonomic nervous tone besides the heart rate. Consideration of the study design, conduct, and type of analyses are important to ensure robust safety and efficacy data are available to guide development of risk-mitigation strategies and regulatory decisions for approval of future clinical trials.

Further studies of ibogaine for medical management of opioid withdrawal and relapse prevention are necessary to fully inform the cardiovascular safety and risk-benefit ratio. In the absence of well-designed studies, the public will face a possible rejection of a potentially beneficial drug for the treatment of opioid use disorder, a condition with high morbidity and mortality. However, based on the current understanding of the cardiac effects of the drug, there will likely be restrictions, including that the drug must be dispensed to patients only in certain health care settings, such as hospitals. In addition, risk-mitigation strategies are necessary to promote its safe use in opioid withdrawal management. These should include medical evaluation before treatment and dynamic electrocardiogram (ECG) monitoring during treatment.

Clinical trials

The FDA first approved an Ibogaine Hydrochloride (Endabuse™) Pharmacokinetics and Pharmacodynamics—Phase I Clinical Trial in May 1993. Following recommendations from the Drug Abuse Advisory Committee (DAAC), which met on 7 April 1995, and the reviewing staff of this Division, a proposed dose escalation study of ibogaine in ibogaine-naive volunteers was approved, under the auspices of an independent data safety monitoring board. The DACC, concerned about dose escalation up to 10 mg.kg, recommended not to exceed the 8 mg/kg used in the original studies of Harris Isbell. Unfortunately, this landmark FDA-approved ibogaine Phase 1 study never progressed owing to a lack of public or private funding.

The UK Medicines and Healthcare Products Regulatory Agency (MHRA) recently granted approval to commence subject enrolment in a Phase 1/2a clinical trial of ibogaine HCl (Eudract Number: 2020-005316-22). QT/QTc measures will be obtained across escalating doses for evaluations that are more precise of ibogaine's proarrhythmic risk before commencing the stage 2 efficacy arm of the study in opioid-dependent patients. Pharmacokinetic (PK) analysis of ibogaine and its metabolite is an integral part of stage 1. Characterization of the pharmacokinetic/pharmacodynamic concentration-response relationship (PK/PD) for QT/QTc prolongation is essential for informing the therapeutic margin of safety of the drug.

Future prospects

Although ibogaine's antiaddictive properties were first widely promoted by Lotsof in 1962, its botanical identification use predates these claims by at least a century. The vast underground experiment of ibogaine as an 'addiction interrupter' is ongoing despite the lack of controlled clinical trials needed for regulatory review of the drug's safety and efficacy. Open-label studies endorse ibogaine as an effective method for managing withdrawal symptoms, affording a transition to abstinence for patients seeking an alternative to long-term opioid substitution therapy. Ibogaine's 'oneiric' state appears to be effective for engaging introspection by giving the patient a focused period to reflect on the negative consequences of drug abuse, while also producing a powerful transformative experience that encourages an awareness of the need to change maladaptive patterns of behaviours. The patient's psychedelic journey with ibogaine seems to help them shift from a precontemplative stage of addiction recovery to a readiness for change. This potential benefit of ibogaine as a psychedelic medicine requires additional study to investigate its use as an adjunct to existing cognitive behavioural or other psychotherapeutic approaches.

The US Centers for Disease Control reported national overdose deaths attributable to opioids and other drugs exceeding 100,000 over a twelve-month period for the first time, despite increased access to medication assisted therapies. The economic cost of the US opioid epidemic in 2017 was estimated at $1,021 billion, including the cost of opioid use disorder estimated at $471 billion and of fatal opioid overdose estimated at $550 billion (Luo & Florence, 2021). The US government and NIDA recently took a significant step towards addressing the opioid crisis by partnering with Delix Therapeutics to study a nonhallucinogenic analogue of ibogaine that may have a better safety profile. More basic pharmacology and nonclinical work still needs to be done to determine if this new molecule has therapeutic effects that are similar to those reported by patients treated with ibogaine. Researchers suggest that the new molecule's psychoplastogen effects may produce sustained therapeutic effects by targeting underlying changes in brain circuitry instead of simply treating the symptoms of the disease (Cameron et al., 2021).

Conclusions

Continued medical research and scientific inquiry into ibogaine as a psychedelic medicine may offer new ways to treat addiction and help confront the opioid crisis. The drug not only helps manage the physical symptoms of withdrawal, cravings, and compulsive drug-seeking but also the behavioural aspects of opioid addiction that drive relapse. The emerging paradigm shift in psychiatry towards use of psychedelic medicines for depression and other mental health disorders may help advance clinical trials of ibogaine and its next generation analogues.

REFERENCES

Alper KR, Beal D, Kaplan CD (2001) A contemporary history of ibogaine in the United States and Europe. The Alkaloids Chemistry and Biology 56:249–281.

Alper, KR, Lotsof, HS, Frenken, GM, et al. (1999) Treatment of acute opioid withdrawal with ibogaine. American Journal of Addictions 8:234–242.

Alper KR, Lotsof HS, Kaplan CD (2008) The ibogaine medical subculture. Journal of Ethnopharmacology 115:9–24.

Antonio T, Childers SR, Rothman RB, et al. (2013) Effect of Iboga alkaloids on mu-opioid receptor coupled G protein activation. PLoS One 8:e77262.

Arias HR, Rosenberg A, Targowska-Duda KM, et al. (2010) Interaction of ibogaine with human alpha3beta4-nicotinic acetylcholine receptors in different conformational states. International Journal of Biochemistry and Cell Biology 42:1525–1535.

Badio B, Padgett WL, Daly JW (1997) Ibogaine: a potent noncompetitive blocker of ganglionic/neuronal nicotinic receptors. Molecular Pharmacology 51:1-5.

Bagal, AA, Hough, LB, Nalwalk, JW, Glick, SD (1996) Modulation of morphine induced antinociception by ibogaine and noribogaine. Brain Research 741:258–262.

Barabe P (1982). Religion of Eboga or the Bwiti of the Fangs. Medecine tropicale: revue du Corps de sante colonial 42:251–257.

Baumann MH, Pablo J, Ali SF, et al. (2001) Comparative neuropharmacology of ibogaine and its O-desmethyl metabolite, noribogaine. The Alkaloids Chemistry and Biology 56:79–113.

Belgers M, Leenaars M, Homberg JR, et al. (2016) Ibogaine and addiction in the animal model, a systematic review and meta-analysis. Translational Psychiatry 6:e826.

Bhargava HN, Cao YJ, Zhao GM (1997) Effects of ibogaine and noribogaine on the antinociceptive action of u-, d-, and k-opioid receptor agonists in mice. Brain Research 752:234–238.

Brown TK, Alper K (2018) Treatment of opioid use disorder with ibogaine: detoxification and drug use outcomes. American Journal of Drug and Alcohol Abuse. 44:24–36.

Bulling S, Schicker K, Zhang YW, et al. (2012) The mechanistic basis for noncompetitive ibogaine inhibition of serotonin and dopamine transporters. Journal of Biological Chemistry 287:18524–18534.

Cameron LP, Tombari RJ, Lu J, et al. (2021) A non-hallucinogenic psychedelic analogue with therapeutic potential. Nature 589:474–479

Camlin TJ, Eulert D, Horvath TA, et al. (2018) A phenomenological investigation into the lived experience of ibogaine and its potential to treat opioid use disorders. Journal of Psychedelic Studies 2018:1–12.

Carnicella S, He DY, Yowell QV, et al. (2010) Noribogaine, but not 18-MC, exhibits similar actions as ibogaine on GDNF expression and ethanol self-administration. Addiction Biology 15:424–433.

Chen K, Kokate TG, Donevan SD, et al. (1996) Ibogaine block of the NMDA receptor: in vitro and in vivo studies. Neuropharmacology 35:423–431.

Codd EE (1995) High affinity ibogaine binding to a mu opioid agonist site. Life Sciences 57:PL315–PL320.

Corkery JM (2018) Ibogaine as a treatment for substance misuse: potential benefits and practical dangers. Progress in Brain Research 242:217–257.

Darke S, Larney S, Farrell M (2017) Yes, people can die from opiate withdrawal. Addiction 112:199–200.

Davis AK, Barsuglia JP, Windham-Herman AM, et al. (2017) Subjective effectiveness of ibogaine treatment for problematic opioid consumption: short—and long-term outcomes and current psychological functioning. Journal of Psychedelic Studies 1:2.

Davis AK, Renn E, Windham-Herman AM, et al. (2018) A Mixed-Method Analysis of Persisting Effects Associated with Positive Outcomes Following Ibogaine Detoxification. Journal of Psychoactive Drugs 50(4):287–297.

Deecher DC, Teitler M, Soderlund DM, et al. (1992) Mechanisms of action of ibogaine and harmaline congeners based on radioligand binding studies. Brain Research 57:242–247.

Destoop M, Morrens M, Coppens V, Dom G (2019) Addiction, anhedonia, and comorbid mood disorder. A narrative review. Frontiers in Psychiatry 10:311.

Dolsen MR, Harvey AG (2017) Life-time history of insomnia and hypersomnia symptoms as correlates of alcohol, cocaine and heroin use and relapse among adults seeking substance use treatment in the United States from 1991 to 1994. Addiction **112**:1104–1111.

Fernandez JW (1982) Bwiti: an ethnography of the religious imagination in Africa: Princeton University Press.

Fernandez JW, Fernandez RL (2001) 'Returning to the path': the use of iboga[ine] in an equatorial African ritual context and the binding of time, space, and social relationships. The Alkaloids Chemistry and Biology **56**:235–247.

Fryer JD, Lukas RJ (1999) Noncompetitive functional inhibition at diverse, human nicotinic acetylcholine receptor subtypes by bupropion, phencyclidine, and ibogaine. Journal of Pharmacology and Experimental Therapeutics **288**:88–92.

Glick SD, Maisonneuve IM, Kitchen BA, Fleck MW (2002) Antagonism of alpha 3 beta 4 nicotinic receptors as a strategy to reduce opioid and stimulant self-administration. European Journal of Pharmacology **438**:99–105.

Glick SD, Maisonneuve IM, Szumlinski KK (2000) 18-Methoxycoronaridine (18-MC) and ibogaine: comparison of antiaddictive efficacy, toxicity, and mechanisms of action. Annals of the New York Academy of Sciences **914**:369–386.

Glue P, Cape G, Tunnicliff D, et al. (2016) Ascending single-dose, double-blind, placebo-controlled safety study of noribogaine in opioid-dependent patients. Clinical Pharmacology in Drug Development **5**:460–468.

Glue P, Winter H, Garbe K, et al. (2015) Influence of CYP2D6 activity on the pharmacokinetics and pharmacodynamics of a single 20 mg dose of ibogaine in healthy volunteers. Journal of Clinical Pharmacology **55**:680–687.

González J, Cavelli M, Castro-Zaballa S, et al. (2021) EEG gamma band alterations and REM-like traits underpin the acute effect of the atypical psychedelic ibogaine in the rat. ACS Pharmacology and Translational Science **4**:517–525.

Goutarel R, Gollnhofer O, Sillans R (1993) Pharmacodynamics and therapeutic applications of iboga and ibogaine. Psychedelic Monographs and Essays **6**:70–111.

Haertzen CA, Meketon MJ (1963) Opiate withdrawal as measured by the Addiction Research Inventory (ARCI). Diseases of the Nervous System **29**:450–455.

Hearn WL, Pablo J, Hime GW, Mash DC (1995) Identification and quantitation of ibogaine and an o-demethylated metabolite in brain and biological fluids using gas chromatography-mass spectrometry. Journal of Analytical Toxicology **19**:427–434.

Helsley S, Filipink RA, Bowen WD, et al. (1998) The effects of sigma, PCP, and opiate receptor ligands in rats trained with ibogaine as a discriminative stimulus. Pharmacology Biochemistry and Behavior **59**:495–503.

Hoffer A, Osmond H (1967) A perceptual hypothesis of schizophrenia. Psychiatry Digest **28**:47–53.

Hough LB, Pearl SM, Glick SD (1996) Tissue distribution of ibogaine after intraperitoneal and subcutaneous administration. Life Sciences **58**:PL119–PL122.

Jacobs MT, Zhang YW, Campbell SD, Rudnick G (2007) Ibogaine, a noncompetitive inhibitor of serotonin transport, acts by stabilizing the cytoplasm-facing state of the transporter. Journal of Biological Chemistry **282**:29441–29447.

Knuijver T, Schellekens A, Belgers M, et al. (2022) Safety of ibogaine administration in detoxification of opioid-dependent individuals: a descriptive open-label observational study. Addiction **117**: 118–128.

Koenig X, Hilber K (2015) The anti-addiction drug ibogaine and the heart: a delicate relation. Molecules 20:2208–2228.

Koenig X, Kovar M, Boehm S, et al. (2014) Anti-addiction drug ibogaine inhibits hERG channels: a cardiac arrhythmia risk. Addiction Biology 19:237–239.

Koob GF, Volkow ND (2010) Neurocircuitry of addiction. Neuropsychopharmacology 35:217–238.

Lambert M, Heckel E (1901) Sur la racine d'Iboga et l'ibogaine. Comptes rendus de l'Académie des Sciences 133:1236–1238.

Lotsof HS (1995) Ibogaine in the treatment of chemical dependency disorders: clinical perspectives. Multidisciplinary Association for Psychedelic Studies 5:16–27.

Luciano D (1998) Observations on treatment with ibogaine. American Journal of Addiction 7:89–90

Luo F, Li M, Florence C (2021) State-level economic costs of opioid use disorder and fatal opioid overdose: United States, 2017. Morbidity and Mortality Weekly Report 70:541–546.

Luz M, Mash DC (2021) Evaluating the toxicity and therapeutic potential of ibogaine in the treatment of chronic opioid abuse. Expert Opinion on Drug Metabolism and Toxicology 17:1019–10122.

Maillet EL, Milon N, Heghinian MD, et al. (2015) Noribogaine is a G-protein biased κ-opioid receptor agonist. Neuropharmacology 99:675–688.

Malik M, Garnett C, Hnatkova K, et al. (2018) Importance of QT/RR hysteresis correction in studies of drug-induced QTc interval changes. Journal of Pharmacokinetics and Pharmacodynamics 45:491–503.

Martin WR, Jasinski DR (1969) Physiological parameters of morphine dependence in man—tolerance, early abstinence, protracted abstinence. Journal of Psychiatric Research 7:9–17.

Mash DC, Ameer B, Prou D, et al. (2016) Oral noribogaine shows high brain uptake and anti-withdrawal effects not associated with place preference in rodents. Journal of Psychopharmacology 30:688–697.

Mash DC, Douyon R, Hearn WL, et al. (1995) A preliminary report on the safety and pharmacokinetics of ibogaine. Biological Psychiatry 9(37):652.

Mash DC, Duque L, Page B, Allen-Ferdinand K (2018) Ibogaine detoxification transitions opioid and cocaine abusers between dependence and abstinence: clinical observations and treatment outcomes. Frontiers in Pharmacology 9:529.

Mash DC, Kovera CA, Buck BE, et al. (1998) Medication development of ibogaine as a pharmacotherapy for drug dependence. Annals of the New York Academy of Sciences 844:274–292

Mash DC, Kovera CA, Pablo J, et al. (2000) Ibogaine: complex pharmacokinetics, concerns for safety, and preliminary efficacy measures. Annals of the New York Academy of Sciences 914:394–401.

Mash DC, Kovera CA, Pablo J, et al. (2001) Ibogaine in the treatment of heroin withdrawal. Alkaloids in Chemistry and Biology 56:155–171.

Mash DC, Staley JK, Baumann MH, et al. (1995) Identification of a primary metabolite of ibogaine that targets serotonin transporters and elevates serotonin. Life Sciences 57:PL45–PL50.

Mash DC, Staley JK, Pablo JP, et al. (1995) Properties of ibogaine and its principal metabolite (12-hydroxyibogamine) at the MK-801 binding site of the NMDA receptor complex. Neuroscience Letters **192**:53–56.

Molinari HH, Maisonneuve IM, Glick SD (1996) Ibogaine neurotoxicity: a re-evaluation. Brain Research **737**:255–262.

Noller GE, Frampton CM, Yazar-Klosinski B (2018) Ibogaine treatment outcomes for opioid dependence from a twelve-month follow-up observational study. American Journal of Drug and Alcohol Abuse **44**:37–46.

Obach RS, Pablo J, Mash DC (1998) Cytochrome P4502D6 catalyzes the O-demethylation of the psychoactive alkaloid ibogaine to 12-hydroxyibogamine. Drug Metabolism and Disposition **25**:1359–1369.

O'Hearn E, Molliver ME (1993) Degeneration of purkinje cells in parasagittal zones of the cerebellar vermis after treatment with ibogaine or harmaline. Neuroscience **55**:303–310.

O'Hearn E, Zhang P, Molliver ME (1995) Excitotoxic insult due to ibogaine leads to delayed induction of neuronal NOS in Purkinje cells. Neuroreport **6**(12):1611–1616.

Olson DE (2018) Psychoplastogens: a promising class of plasticity-promoting neurotherapeutics. Journal of Experimental Neuroscience **12**:1–4.

Pablo JP, Mash DC (1998) Noribogaine stimulates naloxone-sensitive [35S] GTP gammaS binding. Neuroreport **9**:109–114.

Pace CJ, Glick SD, Maisonneuve IM, et al. (2004) Novel iboga alkaloid congeners block nicotinic receptors and reduce drug self-administration. European Journal of Pharmacology **492**:159–167.

Parker LA, Siegel S, Luxton T (1995) Ibogaine attenuates morphine-induced conditioned place preference. Experimental and Clinical Psychopharmacology **3**:344–348.

Pearl SM, Herrick-Davis K, Teitler M, Glick SD (1995) Radioligand-binding study of noribogaine, a likely metabolite of ibogaine. Brain Research **675**:342–344.

Perogamvros L, Schwartz S (2012) The roles of the reward system in sleep and dreaming. Neuroscience and Biobehavioural Reviews **36**:1934–1951.

Phisalix M (1901) Action physiologique de l'ibogaine. Contes Rendu Societe Biologue **53**:1077.

Pope HG (1969) Tabernanthe iboga: an African narcotic plant of social importance. Economic Botany **23**:174–184.

Popik P, Layer RT, Skolnick P (1994) The putative anti-addictive drug ibogaine is competitive inhibitor of [3H]MK-801 binding to the NMDA receptor complex. Psychopharmacology **114**:672–674.

Popik P, Layer RT, Sholnick P (1995) 100 Years of ibogaine: neurochemical and pharmacological actions of a putative anti-addictive drug. Pharmacology Reviews **47**:235–253.

Popik P, Skolnick P (1995) Pharmacology of ibogaine and ibogaine-related alkaloids, in GA Cordell, ed., The alkaloids. Academic Press, 197–231.

Pouchet G, Chevalier J (1905) Les nouveaux remedes. Sur l'action pharmacodynamique de l'ibogaine. Bulletin Géneral de Thérapeutique **149**:211.

Shepard SG (1994) A preliminary investigation of ibogaine: case reports and recommendations for further study. Journal of Substance Abuse Treatment **11**:379–385.

Skolnick P (2001) Ibogaine as a glutamate antagonist: relevance to its putative antiaddictive properties. The Alkaloids Chemistry and Biology 56:55–62.

Skoubis PD, Matthes HW, Walwyn WM, et al. (2001) Naloxone fails to produce conditioned place aversion in mu-opioid receptor knock-out mice. Neuroscience 106:757–763.

Solms M (2000) Dreaming and REM sleep are controlled by different brain mechanisms. Behavioral and Brain Sciences 23:843–850.

Staley JK, Ouyang Q, Pablo J, et al. (1996) Pharmacological screen for activities of 12—hydroxyibogamine: a primary metabolite of the indole alkaloid ibogaine. Psychopharmacology (Berlin) 127:10–18.

Timmermann C, Roseman L, Schartner M, et al. (2019) Neural correlates of the DMT experience assessed with multivariate EEG. Science Reports 9:1–13.

Touchette N (1995) Anti-addiction drug ibogaine on trial. Nature Medicine 1:288–289.

Valentino RJ, Volkow ND (2020) Drugs, sleep, and the addicted brain. Neuropsychopharmacology 45:3–5.

Vicente J, Zusterzeel R, Johannesen L, et al. (2019) Assessment of multi-Ion channel block in a Phase I randomized study design: results of the CiPA Phase I ECG Biomarker Validation Study. Clinical Pharmacology and Therapeutics 105:943–953.

Wells GB, Lopez MC, Tanaka JC, et al. (1999) The effects of ibogaine on dopamine and serotonin transport in rat brain synaptosomes. Brain Research Bulletin 48:641–647.

Zubaran C (2000) Ibogaine and noribogaine: comparing parent compound to metabolite. CNS Drug Reviews 6:219–240.

Zubaran C, Shoaib M, Stolerman IP, et al. (1999) Noribogaine generalization to the ibogaine stimulus: correlation with noribogaine concentration in rat brain. Neuropsychopharmacology 21:119–126.

CHAPTER 8

Other psychedelics

James Linden and Daniel Robin

KEY POINTS

* There are a number of 'lesser-known' psychedelics that have a potential role in treatment of mental health and addictions.
* The agents covered here are magic mushroom–derived muscimol, plant-derived salvinorin A, cactus-derived mescaline, Sasha Shulgin–derived 2C-B, and toad/plant/human–derived 5-methoxy-DMT.
* All these compounds have their unique but overlapping psychedelic effects and side effects.
* Our understanding of plant medicine has the potential to transform much of what we know about psychiatric medicine.

Introduction

This book reviews the current knowledge pertaining to psychedelics and related substances and, in particular, their potential to revolutionize treatment approaches for a range of mental health problems and addictions. This chapter details some of the lesser-known psychedelics (which we henceforward call 'lesser knowns'). While lesser known, some of these are arguably the most potent molecules, and one could argue these hold the most potential for medicine. We go on a small journey into a less-understood corner of plant medicine and psychedelics. Many of the psychedelics discussed so far in this publication have well-elucidated and reasonably well-developed psychopharmacology. The lesser knowns are less understood and have novel effects, the mechanisms underpinning which, are still essentially baffling. In the great pursuit of psychedelic science there has been an increased interest in trying to understand the potential of these lesser-known agents. There are significantly fewer clinical data available for these—in fact none in some cases—at least not of huge or encouraging impact to humanity thus far. It gives great pleasure to present the five lesser knowns shown in Box 8.1.

Muscimol

The widely fabled *Amanita muscaria* (Fly Agaric, AM) mushroom has been revered for centuries by many cultures with relics and folklore emanating from these beautiful red and white mushrooms. AM is arguably the best known entheogenic

> **Box 8.1** 'Lesser-known' psychedelics covered in this chapter
>
> * Magic mushroom–derived muscimol
> * Plant-derived SA
> * Cactus-derived mescaline
> * Sasha Shulgin–derived 2C-B
> * toad/plant/human–derived 5-methoxy-DMT

species on the planet, containing many psychoactive compounds including muscimol and ibotenic acid. Mickey Mouse, Alice in Wonderland, and others have gone on animated adventures revolving around these magical natural phenomena. Some scholars suggest that Santa Claus (Santa Nikalau in Siberia) the Siberian shaman, was visiting families in wintertime with red and white gifts of powerful entheogenic mushrooms. It is argued that these gifts, which grew beside pine trees, give us the Christmas tree culture. Santa Nikalau was said to feed his reindeer the mushrooms, the reindeer would convert the prodrug ibotenic acid, into muscimol through the kidneys. The shaman would then give this muscimol-laced urine to the group he visited. Others have taken this reference of Amanita to Godly levels, believing that Jesus Christ was one such mushroom who was offered by the twelve Apostles—who carried his message to people who were suffering—as the Body of Christ or the Food of the Gods (Soma). While it is hard to learn anything medical or scientific from the God version of the story, the reindeer urine story does make reasonable sense. In modern times, AM is still used for both traditional medicine and for deep soul exploration. This practise is mostly followed in the far Northeast of Europe and Siberia, where the mushroom is most prevalent and grows as a mycorrhizal neighbour to pine trees.

After ingesting the AM mushroom, much of the ibotenic acid is converted to muscimol, through decarboxylation. Often used as a GABA receptor ligand in scientific research, muscimol acts as a very potent selective agonist at the ionotropic GABA receptors, $GABA_A$ and $GABA_C$, and a weak GABA uptake inhibitor (Johnston, 2014). As muscimol binds to the extracellular GABA receptor, the cell's ligand-gated channel opens to allow chloride ions to flow into the neuronal cell, causing a hyperpolarization of charge, making the neuron less likely to generate an action potential and fire. It is for this reason that GABA, the primary inhibitory neurotransmitter of the CNS, reduces neuronal activity and produces the sedative-like effects that make it an attractive drug target for anxiety and convulsions (Phulera et al., 2018).

AM ingestion gives rise to a sense of nausea often overtaken by deep states of euphoric bliss, including level-4 hallucinations, the most intense kind of open-eyed hallucinations. It is widely believed—and has been perpetuated—that AM is toxic once eaten, as there is reportedly a lot of nausea and often vomiting with this mushroom. This could be considered a cleansing purge to those familiar with the commonplace intense vomiting (and less so diarrhoea) associated with ayahuasca consumption (see Chapter 6). One element that makes AM less attractive as an entheogen for modern use is that, to experience the full effects, one must eat the mushroom, digest it, urinate, and then consume the urine. However, the potential to make medicines from this must be reassessed in the modern era, given our new knowledge of the potential mental health benefits of psychedelics, as detailed in other chapters in this book. In particular, muscimol, along with the synthetic drug DOI, are the two psychedelics best known to consistently produce aural hallucinations, which may make it an attractive target for disorders where the patient exhibits auditory symptoms, such as aural hallucinations in people with schizophrenia, and tinnitus, which is associated with a number of medical conditions.

Salvinorin A

Salvia divinorum is a psychedelic plant species which appears to derive from Mexico in Baja California (see review of Casselman et al., 2014). The plant has travelled to, and been successfully propagated, in a host of countries with similar climates. The genome of salvia plants collected across the globe are identical, meaning that no species variation exists for this plant; this is highly unusual. Salvinorin A (SA), the primary active compound, is usually extracted from the plant and concentrated into an oil which is then applied back onto dry leaves of the plant and smoked. This smoking creates an intense psychedelic experience of five to ten minutes in duration.

Unlike many of the classic psychedelics, SA shows no activity at the 5-HT2 receptors, and instead acts as a selective and potent agonist of the κ-opioid receptor (KOR), for which it can attribute its mind-altering effects. SA has shown involvement in the endocannabinoid system as well, likely through cross-functionality of the KOR with the cannabinoid type 1 receptor (Coffeen & Pellicer, 2019). KORs are located throughout the CNS and are implicated in many neurological and behavioural processes such as mood, perception, pain control, stress, and natural reward reinforcement. SA has also been shown experimentally to have an affinity for the dopamine D2 receptor, the primary drug target for antipsychotics (Madras, 2013).

Not only are the genetics of this plant unusual but the compound SA is considered to be the most potent naturally occurring psychedelic (LSD being more potent but part manmade: see Chapter 5): indeed, it is active in micro-g amounts, compared to a relatively hefty 25 mg for a compound like psilocybin (see Chapter 3). SA is also considered by many psychedelic enthusiasts to be somewhat undesirable, as the effects are often negative or at least are perceived as negative at the time of the experience. Many people report two-dimensional hallucinations where the world turns flat and cartoonlike. Others report extreme fear and feelings of wanting to run away or that something is coming after them. These common experiences are at least partially responsible for the scientific community steering exploration towards psychedelic experiences considered to be 'safer', such as psilocybin (Chapter 3) or N,N-DMT (Chapter 6). Because of the rapid onset and equally rapid experience (usually five to ten minutes), it could also be the case that this is too short a time for a counsellor, doctor, or psychiatrist to have any input during the session.

Similar to the issues that Rick Strassman faced with N,N-DMT experiments, there may be a need for infusion or extended-release versions of SA for us to truly explore the potential benefits. Given that it is the most potent natural psychedelic it may make sense for those studying it to explore the efficacy of microdoses. It could be the case that 'a tiny imperceivable bit of something horrible' is just what is required to keep some disorders in check, rather than repeated macrodoses of the negative experience. In Mexico there are groups who ingest the plant and work with it over a longer period, but the amount of scientific data on this is very slim. There are those salvia enthusiasts who argue that the darker threads of salvia trips are an integral requirement of fully resolving shadow issues that the lighter and fluffier psychedelics simply don't touch.

Mescaline

Mescaline is produced by a number of species of cactus, and the cacti are known to have been used for almost six millennia by Native American tribes in Rio Grande, Texas. It could be argued that mescaline is the longest human-use psychedelic, where its consumption was not by accident or through the ingestion of a range of foraged fungi: rather, it was known for its entheogenic powers and was deliberately sought out. It is possible that the use of magic mushrooms and entheogens by druids in Western Europe (particularly in Ireland) dates further back, but there is no clear evidence to truly determine this beyond some pouches found with psilocybin mushrooms and similar findings in burial chambers (see also Chapter 1).

Mescaline remains widely utilized by the indigenous cultures who grow and consume the cacti that produce it, as well as by those who visit retreats, mainly in Central and South America. The psychedelic cacti community work with a number of cacti species. Peyote grows naturally in the southern United States and in the deserts of Mexico where it is probably best known. In the Amazon regions the most popular cactus is San Pedro, which grows easily and has been cultivated in other parts of the world with little effort. The least-known and least-discussed cactus is the Peruvian torch, which is a relative of San Pedro that grows in the high Andean plains. While San Pedro is common and grows easily, Peyote has been severely overharvested in its natural environment. The cultivation and extraction of mescaline from cacti could prove extremely efficient because of the nature of the base material itself, which makes extractions relatively straightforward.

Mescaline is a phenethylamine, whereas psilocybin and N,N-DMT are tryptamines (like serotonin and melatonin). Psychedelics master chemist Alexander Sasha Shulgin based a number of novel compounds on mescaline's benzene ring structure. In his book PIHKAL, he details dozens of these molecules that he and his wife trialled themselves over a period of some forty years (reviewed by Gems, 1999). Noted for being the godfather of the MDMA emergence, Sasha Shulgin didn't actually create MDMA, but he did create two very well-known psychedelics that are known by the dance music world and across the psychedelic community: 2CI and 2C-B, which are essentially mescaline with an iodine or bromine group substituted on the second carbon of the benzene ring. The effects are profoundly different between mescaline, 2CI, and 2C-B, and similarly for the other analogues he created.

Mescaline is a serotonergic partial agonist that depends on the glutamatergic cortical network for its psychedelic mechanism of action. It does so by binding with high affinity to the 5-HT$_{2A}$ receptors in the deep cortical layers and prefrontal cortex, in turn increasing spontaneity in glutamatergic activity and the willingness of neurons to communicate (Béïque, et al., 2007). This causes a disruption in the normal 'rhythmic oscillation' in the neural system and increases entropy throughout the brain. This process results in an increase in synaptic plasticity in the cortex and is also purported to be responsible for the altered state of consciousness seen with serotonin 5-HT$_{2A}$ agonist psychedelics.

Mescaline generally offers a warm and caring empathic feeling, similar to what someone using LSD and MDMA together would experience. It generates interesting empathic effects at low to high doses, along with some intense hallucinations at doses over 500 milligrams (high dose). Indeed, at higher doses it is a very powerful and extremely long-lasting psychedelic (up to twenty hours). Users experience euphoria and deep introspection often accompanied by some vomiting and purging. The long duration of action of mescaline has been an impediment to clinical research. Even in small doses the effects last four to six hours and come without a true 'breakthrough' experience.

2C-B

2C-B is a fast-acting, medium-duration (~4 hours) phenethylamine. Unlike its phenethylamine cousin mescaline, 2C-B induces little activity at the 5-HT$_{2A}$ and 5-HT$_{2C}$ receptors, indicating it to be a partial 5-HT agonist at best (Gonzalez et al., 2015). Conversely, some studies have shown that 2C-B acts as a potent inhibitor of the serotonin transporter (SERT) protein in a similar manner to MDMA, making it a serotonergic antagonist that is mechanistically comparable to an SRI (Montgomery et al., 2007). Like other phenethylamines and tryptamines, 2-CB has a high affinity at the trace-amine receptor, implicated in the emotional and sensory centres of the brain.

2C-B has been used by partygoers and consciousness explorers since Sasha Shulgin released it circa 1990. Like its counterpart, 2CI, it can produce profound hallucinations for a period of three to six hours, dose dependent. The pure form of the drug, when taken on its own, is considered to be relatively safe and has no recorded fatalities attributed to it. 2C-B has emerged as a strong candidate for promotion into clinical settings. The usually controllable nature of the trip means that a user who is experiencing a bad trip can simply open their eyes to control the distressing effects. This allows the user to grasp a small window on reality which can be deeply reassuring during an intense experience.

Sasha Shulgin suggested that while MDMA and mescaline are empathogenic, if there was ever a drug discovered that represented the feeling of love, its effects would equate to that of 2C-B, or something very close. There is currently a raft of pharmaceutical companies turning their interest towards novel psychedelics and novel psychedelic analogues (see Chapter 11). It appears that minor changes to structure can totally alter the drug profile. The library created by Sasha Shulgin alone can provide the basis for decades of exploration and refinement.

5-MeO-DMT

We complete this chapter by paying some attention to what many feel is the most interesting and most powerful psychedelic of them all. It gives us great pleasure to introduce 5-methoxy-N,N-DMT (5-MeO), aka the 'God Molecule'.

5-MeO is an extremely powerful, naturally occurring, psychedelic tryptamine from the same class as psilocybin and N,N-DMT. Other important tryptamines are the endogenous ones which were previously mentioned, such as serotonin, melatonin, N,N-DMT, and bufotenine. 5-MeO is also believed to be endogenous in humans as a transient neurotransmitter, but there has been no definitive study to prove this. The role of the compound is as yet entirely unknown, but it seems likely that it is involved in standard brain function.

5-MeO is a nonselective serotonergic receptor agonist that inhibits serotonin reuptake with an affinity for a range of 5-HT, norepinephrine, sigma, dopamine, and other receptor sites. 5-MeO binds with highest affinity to the 5-HT_{1A} receptor subtype, and to a lesser extent, the 5-HT_{2A} and 5-HT_{2C} receptors (Krebs-Thompson et al., 2006). Activation at the 5-HT_{1A} receptor, located throughout the limbic system, reduces the cell firing rate in the dorsal raphe nucleus and promotes dopamine release in the hippocampus, striatum, and medial prefrontal cortex (Heidenreich et al., 1989). 5-MeO also interacts with the trace-amine receptor system. 5-MeO is primarily metabolized by MAO A, but it is also partially converted into 5-HO-DMT (bufotenine), another endogenous psychedelic compound, which has a higher binding affinity to 5-HT_{2A} than 5-MeO.

5-MeO is an experience like nothing else. Usually smoked, upon inhalation, one dissolves into the cosmos and joins the great oneness. One could try for days to describe this more scientifically, but those words do not yet exist. This compound does not usually produce beautiful fractal geometric hallucinations or visual distortions into comical caricatures as with other psychedelics. Rather, the experience is more of a heavy body load with inconsistent trip experiences that range from becoming an animal in the jungle through to reliving trauma from childhood through to visiting or speaking to dead relatives.

In the 1960s there was huge interest in this molecule. As the duration of the associated trip is between ten to forty minutes, it makes an ideal tool for psychiatry and psychotherapy to work alongside, whereas psilocybin and ayahuasca last for many hours, which is a hugely expensive cost for staffing. Ralph Metzner was the true leader in this field. He worked with 5-MeO in the 1960s and created foundations for new companies to uncover the mysteries around how these drugs work.

Around 1983 an American traveller in Mexico, Ken Nelson, is credited with the first documented case of smoking 5-MeO, in this case taken from the venom of the Sonoran Desert toad, *Bufo alvarius*. The journey was intense and was immediately immortalized, and this catalysed a new craze for smoking 'toad medicine'. Various tribes in north Mexico, the Siri tribe for one, have been developing working methods for the administration of toad venom to drug addicts. Around 2010, Mexican doctor Octavio Rettig began working with drug addicts in Sonora where large populations of crystal methamphetamine and crack cocaine addicts have become commonplace. He has given treatments to over 10,000 people across the world who have struggled with addiction or trauma or who have been seeking spiritual exploration. The results have been impressive, and a number of emerging psychedelic entities are shifting their attention to 5-MeO as an antiaddictive agent, while some have focused their attention on the trauma-relieving elements and possible potential as an antidepressant (see Ermakova et al., 2021). Clearly much more work is required to determine efficacy and safety of 5-MeO, but the potential to address severe addictive disorders is enormously exciting.

Conclusions

The psychedelic renaissance is producing many new rising stars who can carry the mantle for the great psychedelic researchers like Albert Hofmann, Sasha Shulgin, and Ralph Metzner, to help us fully elucidate the potential for the plethora of psychedelic drugs that could and already are transforming medicine.

REFERENCES

Béïque JC, Imad M, Mladenovic L, et al. (2007) Mechanism of the 5-hydroxytryptamine 2A receptor-mediated facilitation of synaptic activity in prefrontal cortex. Proceedings of the National Academy of Sciences 104:9870–9875.

Casselman I, Nock CJ, Wohlmuth H, et al. (2014) From local to global—fifty years of research on *Salvia divinorum*. Journal of Ethnopharmacology 151:768–783.

Coffeen U, Pellicer F (2019) *Salvia divinorum*: from recreational hallucinogenic use to analgesic and anti-inflammatory action. Journal of Pain Research 12:1069–1076

El-Seedi HR, De Smet PA, Beck O et al. (2005). Prehistoric peyote use: alkaloid analysis and radiocarbon dating of archaeological specimens of Lophophora from Texas. Journal of Ethnopharmacology 101:238–242.

Ermakova AO, Dunbar F, Rucker J, Johnson MW (2021) A narrative synthesis of research with 5-MeO-DMT. Journal of Psychopharmacology 36(3):273–294. 02698811211050543.

Gems D (1999) Alexander Shulgin and Ann Shulgin, PIHKAL, a chemical love story. Alexander Shulgin and Ann Shulgin, TIHKAL, the continuation. Theoretical Medicine and Bioethics **20**:477–479.

González D, Torrens M, Farré M (2015) Acute effects of the novel psychoactive drug 2C-B on emotions. BioMed Research International 1–9:643878.

Heidenreich BA, Rebec GV (1989) Serotonergic dorsal raphe neurons: changes in spontaneous neuronal activity and responsiveness to 5-MeODMT following long-term amphetamine administration. Neuroscience Letters **103**:81–86.

Johnston GAR (2014) Muscimol as an ionotropic GABA receptor agonist. Neurochemical Research **39**:1942–1947.

Krebs-Thomson K, Ruiz EM, Masten V, et al. (2006) The roles of 5-HT1A and 5-HT2 receptors in the effects of 5-MeO-DMT on locomotor activity and prepulse inhibition in rats. Psychopharmacology **189**:319–329.

Madras B (2013) History of the discovery of the antipsychotic dopamine d2 receptor: a basis for the dopamine hypothesis of schizophrenia. Journal of the History of the Neurosciences **22**:62–78.

Montgomery T, Buon C, Eibauer S et al. (2007) Comparative potencies of 3,4-methylenedioxymethamphetamine (MDMA) analogues as inhibitors of [3H] noradrenaline and [3H]5-HT transport in mammalian cell lines. British Journal of Pharmacology **152**:1121–1130.

Nichols DE (2004) Hallucinogens. Pharmacology and Therapeutics **101**:131–181.

Phulera S, Zhu H, Yu J, et al. (2018) Cryo-EM structure of the benzodiazepine-sensitive α1β1γ2S tri-heteromeric GABAA receptor in complex with GABA. Elife **7**:e39383.

CHAPTER 8

CHAPTER 9

Ketamine

Joshua D. Di Vincenzo, Joshua D. Rosenblat, and
Roger S. McIntyre

KEY POINTS

* Ketamine, at subanaesthetic doses, is a safe, rapid-acting, and significantly
  effective antidepressant in patients with treatment-resistant depression (TRD).
* Evidence also suggests that ketamine is effective at reducing suicidal ideation.
* Ketamine is the first glutamatergic agent that is Food and Drug Administration
  (FDA) approved in depression treatment.
* Ketamine's mechanism of action is still being ascertained.

Ketamine is a racemate of two enantiomers referred to as (R)-ketamine and
(S)-ketamine, or arketamine and esketamine. Developed as a derivative of the
anaesthetic drug phencyclidine (PCP) with fewer adverse effects and lower
abuse potential, ketamine has been commercially available for five decades and
widely used in anaesthesia since 1970. Unlike most psychedelics, which elicit
their subjective effects by activating *serotonergic* 5-HT2a receptors, ketamine
mainly targets *glutamatergic* systems and is therefore not considered a 'classic
psychedelic'. Instead, ketamine is more commonly referred to as a dissociative
anaesthetic, although it is gaining prominence outside of anaesthesia for its capacity to treat treatment-resistant depression (TRD; i.e. inadequate response to
≥ 2 antidepressants of different classes within a current depressive episode) and
suicidality. It is included in this book for reasons articulated in the preface.

Psychopharmacology of ketamine

The pharmacology of ketamine is complicated because of its racemic nature and
convoluted metabolic pathway as it is converted to various active metabolites.
Ketamine possesses its highest binding affinity (K_i = 0.25 micromolar) at exci-
tatory glutamatergic N-methyl D-aspartate receptors (NMDARs) in the central
nervous system (CNS), where the drug binds to the allosteric PCP site within the
channel pore and acts as a non-competitive open channel blocker (Zanos et al.,
2018). Because of its lipophilicity, ketamine has significant bioavailability through
various routes of administration, readily crosses the blood-brain barrier, and it
reaches the CNS within one minute following intravenous (IV) administration

and/or entry into the bloodstream. The oral bioavailability of racemic keta-mine is 20%–30%, owing to extensive first-pass metabolism, with peak concen-trations (C_{max}) occurring between 20 and 120 minutes (Yanagihara et al., 2003). Interestingly, esketamine has a significantly lower oral bioavailability (~10%) com-pared to racemic ketamine or arketamine because stereoselective cytochrome p450 (CYP)-3A4 enzymes involved in the first-pass effect possess a greater af-finity for the S-enantiomer compared to the R-enantiomer (Fanta et al., 2015; Portmann et al., 2010). Intranasal administration circumvents the first-pass effect, with a bioavailability of approximately 50%, making it preferred over the oral route for esketamine delivery (Yanagihara et al., 2003).

At therapeutic concentrations, ketamine is largely metabolized to norketamine, an active metabolite which inhibits α7nACh nicotinic acetylcholine receptors at nanomolar concentrations (Moaddel et al., 2013). Norketamine is measurable in the plasma within three minutes of IV ketamine administration and reaches C_{max} at approximately thirty minutes (Mion & Villevieille, 2013). Norketamine is subse-quently metabolized into hydroxynorketamine (HNK) and dehydronorketamine, both of which are also α7nACh receptor inhibitors at nanomolar concentrations (Moaddel et al., 2013). A subanaesthetic IV dose of ketamine resulted in a HNK C_{max} approximately 1/10th the magnitude of the C_{max} of ketamine, which oc-curred at approximately four hours postdose; however, the overall exposure (area under the curve) of HNK was greater than that of ketamine (Zarate et al., 2012). The significant exposures and pharmacological activities of ketamine's metabolites may help explain its protracted effects on mood, which persist even after the drug is cleared from the body.

Effects on the brain

Ketamine's mechanism of action is thought to involve targeting molecular systems that initiate a cascade of events with consequent effects on cortico-limbic brain regions. Cortico-limbic dysfunction is central to the aetiopathogenesis of major depressive disorder (MDD) and other psychiatric disorders, and ketamine has been found to modulate cortico-limbic brain regions in ways which may normalize this dysfunction. Many of the proposed mechanisms of action of ketamine have been summarized in a review by Zanos and Gould (2018), including five of the most prominent, which are shown in Box 9.1. Importantly, these mechanisms are not mutually exclusive and likely act in synergy.

Studies involving neuroimaging are advancing our understanding of ketamine's effects on the brain (see Ionescu et al., (2018) for a review on neuroimaging studies of ketamine). For example, it has been established that ketamine admin-istration leads to a short-term increase in local glutamate signalling within the prefrontal cortex (PFC), a brain region whose dysfunction is highly implicated in depression. This rapid glutamatergic activation may induce long-term potenti-ation, offering another possible mechanism by which the antidepressant effects of ketamine can be sustained after the drug has been cleared from the body.

Box 9.1 Five commonly proposed mechanisms of action of ketamine's antidepressant effects on cortico-limbic circuits

1. Disinhibition of glutamate release at pyramidal neurons by blockade of NMDARs on inhibitory GABAergic interneurons, leading to brain-derived neurotrophic factor (BDNF) release, activation of the tropomyosin receptor kinase B (TrkB) receptor and promotion of protein synthesis via activation of the mechanistic target of rapamycin complex 1 (mTORC1)

2. Blockade of extra-synaptic NMDARs, which, under basal conditions inhibit protein synthesis via the mTOR pathway, leading to desuppression of protein synthesis

3. Blockade of spontaneous NMDAR activity at the postsynaptic neuron, inhibiting elongation factor 2 kinase (eEF2K) activity, leading to upregulation of BDNF translation

4. Metabolites of ketamine, like HNK, acting on NMDAR-independent pathways, such as promoting α-amino-3-hydroxy-5-methyl-4-isoxazolepropionic acid receptor (AMPAR)-mediated synaptic potentiation

5. Attenuation of excessive NMDAR-dependent burst firing of neurons in the lateral habenula, a brain region that shows consistent overactivity in depression

Adapted with permission from Zanos P, Gould TD. Mechanisms of ketamine action as an antidepressant. Molecular Psychiatry 23(4):801–811. Copyright © 2018 Springer Nature.

Moreover, ketamine facilitates changes in functional connectivity between brain regions. Evidence suggests that ketamine may decrease functional connectivity between the dorsal and pregenual regions of the anterior cingulate cortex, and between the default mode network and PFC; two circuits involved in ruminative thinking. Hence, the modulation of neural circuits underlying maladaptive behaviours or thought patterns such as rumination provides yet another mechanism by which ketamine effects the brain. Interestingly, unlike therapy with classic psychedelics (see Chapters 3, 5, and 6) and MDMA (Chapter 4), wherein the 'trip' experience is purported to be an essential constituent of treatment through which therapeutic insights are derived, the 'trip' or dissociation experienced during ketamine therapy is considered a side effect of the drug. While dissociation severity has largely been orthogonal to improvement in depression with ketamine, Clinician-Administered Dissociative States Scale (CADSS) scores may correlate with antidepressant response (Luckenbaugh et al., 2014), but this has not been ascertained in randomized controlled trials (RCTs). Furthermore, the CADSS does not appear to adequately capture the psychoactive effects of ketamine (Van Schalkwyk et al., 2018), highlighting the need for a more appropriate rating scale, incorporating components of mysticism, by which to assess dissociation in ketamine therapy. Thus, ketamine exerts many effects on disparate brain regions, which likely act together to ameliorate depressive symptomatology.

Clinical evidence

Shortly after being marketed as an anaesthetic in the 1970s, clinicians began to notice and study the 'mind-expanding' potential of ketamine at *subanaesthetic* doses. In the first ever study of ketamine in psychiatry, Khorramzadeh and Lotfy (1973) reported mostly positive outcomes in one hundred psychiatric inpatients in Iran with various diagnoses, treated with subanaesthetic doses of ketamine. However, the study of ketamine in psychiatry was not prioritized until more recently. Since the advent of the RCT as the gold standard for evaluating pharmacotherapies, ketamine has been rigorously studied in numerous RCTs and real-world, open-label settings. In 2000, the first RCT ($n = 7$) of IV ketamine for depression was published, showing 0.5 mg/kg of racemic ketamine to be superior to placebo, with peak antidepressant effects reported after seventy-two hours (Berman et al., 2000). This encouraging pilot study spurred on several RCTs seeking to replicate these findings in larger populations of individuals with bipolar disorder (BD) and TRD, wherein response rates exceeding 60% were reported following single doses of ketamine, compared to < 30% following midazolam control (Diazgranados et al., 2010; Murrough et al., 2013; Zarate et al., 2006). These studies also provided insights into the duration of ketamine's antidepressant effects, which tend to emerge within hours of administration and gradually subside within a week as depressive symptoms return. Subsequent studies found that additional doses of ketamine (a.k.a. 'boosters') could safely prolong the antidepressant effects elicited by a single dose and prevent relapse (aan het Rot et al., 2010; Murrough et al., 2013), leading to the widespread adoption of repeated-dosing regimens of ketamine to treat depression.

Since the year 2000, the number of studies published per year on PubMed with the keywords 'ketamine' and 'depression' has increased twenty-fold, and it has become more common in certain jurisdictions for psychiatrists to prescribe off-label ketamine in various formulations (e.g. IV ketamine, intranasal esketamine, and oral ketamine) to treat TRD and suicidality. These developments set the stage for regulatory approval. In 2019, based on replicated clinical trials, Spravato® esketamine nasal spray was approved with fast-track and breakthrough designations by the FDA, adjunct to an oral antidepressant, for the treatment of TRD and suicidality—the first FDA approval of a ketamine product for a psychiatric indication. Today, various formulations of ketamine have been studied in thousands of participants both within clinical trials and naturalistic settings, providing sufficient data to enable meta-analyses. In a recent meta-analysis, the pooled effect size of IV, intranasal, and oral ketamine or esketamine administration on reducing depressive symptomatology was moderate and significant, Hedges' $g = 0.529$ (N = 31 studies, pooled sample size = 1452 participants, 95% confidence interval: 0.328 to 0.729, $p < 0.01$) across all time points from twenty-four hours to twenty-eight days postdose, with moderate heterogeneity ($p < 0.01$, $I^2 = 50.38\%$) (McIntyre et al., 2020). Another recent meta-analysis investigated the effect of ketamine on reducing suicidal ideation, and reported a large and

> **Box 9.2** Convergent findings of clinical trials on ketamine in psychiatry
>
> * 0.5mg/kg appears to be the minimum effective dose, and most tolerable at which to initiate treatment with IV ketamine
> * Transient dissociation, nausea, hypertension, and anxiety are the most commonly reported treatment-emergent adverse events
> * Significant positive effects on mood are often observed within hours of a single dose, and may persist for multiple days or weeks
> * Booster or repeated ketamine doses are safe and effective at preventing and/or treating the re-emergence of depressive symptoms following a first dose

significant pooled effect size of Hedges' $g = 1.029$ (N = 9, pooled sample size = 197, 95% CI: 0.748 to 1.310, $p < 0.001$) across all formulations and routes and time points, up to 24 hours after dosing, with significant heterogeneity ($p < 0.05$, $I^2 = 56.82\%$) (Xiong et al., 2021). There is evidence of differing efficacy and patterns of response between formulations/routes of administration (i.e. timing of peak antidepressant effect after treatment); however, comparisons could not be made because of heterogeneity. Thus, adequately powered, head-to-head trials are needed to investigate the potential differences in tolerability and effectiveness of disparate ketamine formulations and routes of administration. Interestingly, both early and recent clinical trials of ketamine for depression have converged on several key findings, as shown in Box 9.2.

Suggestions for clinical use

Many of the safety concerns associated with recreational ketamine use (e.g. urological disorders, addiction or craving) have not been replicated within the context of psychiatry. Although treatment-emergent adverse events (TEAEs) are reported frequently, they are mostly acceptable and do not constitute a major barrier to the implementation of ketamine therapy: only 1%–5% of participants discontinue use because of safety or tolerability issues in clinical trials. Evidence from clinical trials and real-world settings suggests most TEAEs are benign and transient, with onset and peak occurring within two hours, and spontaneous resolution within twenty-four hours postdose. In esketamine trials, patients who experienced severe TEAEs were more likely to weigh more, be female, receive antidepressant polypharmacy, and receive a higher esketamine dose. Thus, patient selection is a critical juncture at which TEAEs can be mitigated. Importantly, weight gain and sexual dysfunction, the most commonly cited reasons for nonadherence to monoaminergic antidepressants, are not observed with ketamine. Table 9.1 summarizes five of the most common TEAEs associated with ketamine in psychiatry, with prevention and management strategies offered for each.

Table 9.1 Common adverse events associated with ketamine and esketamine, with applicable prevention and management strategies

Adverse event	Overview	Prevention	Management[a]
Dissociation	State of altered consciousness involving a subjective feeling of disconnection from one's environment and/or self; peaks within 40 min, usually resolves within 1–2 h postadministration; may elicit a negative or positive subjective experience; not clinically significant in the majority of patients; likely dose dependent; intensity and incidence diminish with repeated infusions.	Patient education; create an environment that feels safe, comfortable, and is not overly stimulating (e.g. quiet dimly lit room, can provide blankets); play calming music or encourage patients to create a personal playlist; baseline psychiatric assessment; support patients to begin treatment in a calm and relaxed mindset as pre-existing distress or agitation may be exacerbated.	**Assessment:** CADSS-6 Mental health professionals should be available to assist with patient distress. **Pharmacological interventions**:** Benzodiazepines*, atypical antipsychotics, and antihistamines. *May increase sedation and interfere with treatment response. **Not recommended except in severe cases.
Anxiety	The most commonly reported psychiatric TEAE; usually dissipates within 2 h postadministration.	Patient education; create an environment that feels safe, comfortable, and is not overly stimulating (e.g. quiet dimly lit room, can provide blankets); play calming music, or encourage patients to create a personal playlist; baseline psychiatric assessment; support patients to begin treatment in a calm and relaxed mindset as pre-existing distress or agitation may be exacerbated.	**Assessment:** GAD-7 Mental health professional should be available to assist with patient distress; Breathing and mindfulness exercises, can apply a cold compress to the back of the neck. **Pharmacological interventions**:** Benzodiazepines*, atypical antipsychotics and antihistamines. *May increase sedation and interfere with ketamine/esketamine response. **Not recommended except in severe cases.

Table 9.1 Continued

Adverse event	Overview	Prevention	Management[a]
Increased blood pressure	Elevations in systolic and diastolic blood pressure of 10%–50%; observed within 30–50 min postadministration and normalize within 2–4 h; individuals with pre-existing conditions (e.g. hypertension, diabetes mellitus) may exhibit greater blood pressure increases and may be more prone to clinically significant hypertension.	Clinical management of pre-existing hypertension and related cardiovascular and metabolic conditions; blood pressure should be measured pretreatment, throughout the treatment (i.e. at 40 min following administration), and for at least 2 h following administration until values normalize.	Trained nurse or clinician should be available to manage hypertension. **Pharmacological interventions:** Clinically significant cases may necessitate antihypertensive treatment such as beta-blockers (e.g. labetalol, metoprolol), vasodilators (e.g. hydralazine), calcium channel blockers (e.g. amlodipine), and/or alpha-adrenergic agonists (e.g. clonidine); at least one care provider should have ACLS training.
Nausea	May be dose dependent; incidence and intensity diminish with repeated treatment; may be more common amongst female patients.	Patients should undergo a fasting period of 2 h prior to intranasal esketamine treatment and 6–8 h prior to ketamine infusion; a prolonged fasting period and/or prophylactic antiemetics may be warranted during subsequent treatments for patients reporting severe nausea during the first treatment; pre-existing GERD may exacerbate nausea and should be treated before ketamine or esketamine administration.	Breathing and mindfulness exercises, can apply cold compress to the back of the neck. **Pharmacological interventions:** Antiemetics (e.g. ondansetron, dimenhydrinate).
Headache	Typically resolves within 1–4 h postadministration.	Creating an environment that feels safe, comfortable, and is not overly stimulating (e.g. quiet dimly lit room, can provide blankets); play calming music or encourage patients to create a personal playlist.	Breathing and mindfulness exercises. **Pharmacological interventions:** Over-the-counter analgesics* (e.g. acetaminophen). *NSAIDs may worsen gastric irritation and are thus not recommended.

ACLS = advanced cardiovascular life support; CADSS-6 = Clinician-Administered Dissociative States 6-Item Scale; GAD-7 = Generalized Anxiety Disorder 7-Item Scale; GERD = gastroesophageal reflux disease; mmHg = millimetre of mercury; NSAID = nonsteroidal anti-inflammatory drug; TEAE = treatment-emergent adverse event.

[a] IV pharmacological interventions are only recommended for adverse effects of IV ketamine wherein an IV line has been pre-established.

Adapted with permission from Ceban et al. (2021) Prevention and management of common adverse effects of ketamine and esketamine in patients with mood disorders. CNS Drugs 35:925–934. Copyright © 2021 Springer Nature.

Conclusions

Ketamine is a safe and efficacious tool for treating TRD and suicidality. Ketamine is often considered a psychedelic because of the subjective dissociative state it evokes, despite the significant differences in pharmacology and implementation between ketamine and serotonergic agents like psilocybin (Chapter 3) and LSD (Chapter 5). Some of the main advantages of ketamine, compared to current first-line antidepressants, include the absence of adverse effects relating to sexual dysfunction and weight gain, rapid onset of action, and efficacy in treatment-resistant individuals. However, ketamine is currently reserved for treatment-resistant cases of depression, is most often prescribed adjunct to monoaminergic antidepressants, and treatment sessions require monitoring by trained personnel. In addition to elucidating its mechanism(s) of action, further research is needed to determine whether ketamine is a safe and effective first-line treatment or monotherapy for depression, and to determine efficacy in the long-term, as well as across other mental disorders (e.g., bipolar disorder).

Future directions

While ketamine may be further along in the clinical trials/regulatory approval pipeline compared to classic psychedelics, there remains much to learn and the mechanisms underlying ketamine's antidepressant effects are still under investigation (see McIntyre et al., 2021 for a comprehensive discussion of future directions). Neuroimaging studies should continue to yield valuable insights on these mechanisms, as well as the aetiopathogenesis of depression. The increasing availability of clinical data and emergence of pharmacogenomics have enabled studies on predictors of antidepressant response based on patient characteristics (e.g. body-mass index, CYP polymorphisms, and clinical features). However, currently, predictive models are not yet robust enough to be clinically useful, which warrants continued investigation. Additionally, the majority of clinical trials have investigated ketamine adjunct to oral antidepressants; therefore, our understanding of ketamine as a monotherapy for depression is still nascent. Head-to-head RCTs comparing ketamine monotherapy and adjunctive therapy are required to determine whether ketamine could feasibly be prescribed as monotherapy to avoid polypharmacy and mitigate side effect burden. Moreover, some smaller studies have hinted at the potential of ketamine to treat other psychiatric conditions such as substance use disorders, posttraumatic stress disorder, and obsessive-compulsive disorder, but high-quality evidence for these indications is scant, and larger studies are required. Furthermore, arketamine and esketamine exhibit different pharmacokinetics and pharmacodynamics, which may be clinically relevant (see Chapter 11). Head-to-head trials comparing different ketamine formulations and routes of administration are required to optimize treatment regimens.

REFERENCES

aan het Rot M, Collins KA, Murrough JW, et al. (2010) Safety and efficacy of repeated-dose intravenous ketamine for treatment-resistant depression. Biological Psychiatry 67:139–145.

Berman RM, Cappiello A, Anand A, et al. (2000) Antidepressant effects of ketamine in depressed patients. Biological Psychiatry 47:351–354.

Ceban F, Rosenblat JD, Kratiuk K, et al. (2021) Prevention and management of common adverse effects of ketamine and esketamine in patients with mood disorders. CNS Drugs 35:925–934.

Diazgranados N, Ibrahim L, Brutsche NE, et al. (2010) A randomized add-on trial of an N-methyl-D-aspartate antagonist in treatment-resistant bipolar depression. Archives of General Psychiatry 67:793–802.

Fanta S, Kinnunen M, Backman JT, Kalso E (2015) Population pharmacokinetics of S-ketamine and norketamine in healthy volunteers after intravenous and oral dosing. European Journal of Clinical Pharmacology 71:441–447.

Ionescu DF, Felicione JM, Gosai A, et al. (2018) Ketamine-associated brain changes: a review of the neuroimaging literature. Harvard Review of Psychiatry 26:320–339.

Khorramzadeh E, Lotfy AO (1973) The use of ketamine in psychiatry. Psychosomatics 14:344–346.

Luckenbaugh DA, Niciu MJ, Ionescu DF, et al. (2014) Do the dissociative side effects of ketamine mediate its antidepressant effects? Journal of Affective Disorders 159:56.

McIntyre RS, Carvalho IP, Lui LMW, et al. (2020) The effect of intravenous, intranasal, and oral ketamine in mood disorders: a meta-analysis. Journal of Affective Disorders 276:576–584.

McIntyre RS, Rosenblat JD, Nemeroff CB, et al. (2021) Synthesizing the evidence for ketamine and esketamine in treatment-resistant depression: an international expert opinion on the available evidence and implementation. American Journal of Psychiatry 178(5):383–399. doi:10.1176/appi.ajp.2020.20081251.

Mion G, Villevieille T (2013) Ketamine pharmacology: an update (pharmacodynamics and molecular aspects, recent findings). CNS Neuroscience and Therapeutics 19:370–380.

Moaddel R, Abdrakhmanova G, Kozak J, et al. (2013) Sub-anesthetic concentrations of (R,S)-ketamine metabolites inhibit acetylcholine-evoked currents in α7 nicotinic acetylcholine receptors. European Journal of Pharmacology 698:228.

Murrough JW, Iosifescu DV, Chang LC, et al. (2013) Antidepressant efficacy of ketamine in treatment-resistant major depression: a two-site randomized controlled trial. American Journal of Psychiatry 170:1134–1142.

Murrough JW, Perez AM, Pillemer S, et al. (2013) Rapid and longer-term antidepressant effects of repeated ketamine infusions in treatment-resistant major depression. Biological Psychiatry 74:250–256.

Portmann S, Kwan HY, Theurillat R, et al. (2010) Enantioselective capillary electrophoresis for identification and characterization of human cytochrome P450 enzymes which metabolize ketamine and norketamine in vitro. Journal of Chromatography A 1217:7942–7948.

Van Schalkwyk GI, Wilkinson ST, Davidson L, et al. (2018) Acute psychoactive effects of intravenous ketamine during treatment of mood disorders: analysis of the Clinician Administered Dissociative State Scale. Journal of Affective Disorders **227**:11.

Xiong J, Lipsitz O, Chen-Li D, Rosenblat JD, et al. (2021) The acute antisuicidal effects of single-dose intravenous ketamine and intranasal esketamine in individuals with major depression and bipolar disorders: a systematic review and meta-analysis. Journal of Psychiatric Research **134**:57–68.

Yanagihara Y, Ohtani M, Kariya S, et al. (2003) Plasma concentration profiles of ketamine and norketamine after administration of various ketamine preparations to healthy Japanese volunteers. Biopharmaceutics and Drug Disposition **24**:37–43.

Zanos P, Gould TD (2018) Mechanisms of ketamine action as an antidepressant. Molecular Psychiatry **23**:801–811.

Zanos P, Moaddel R, Morris PJ, et al. (2018) Ketamine and ketamine metabolite pharmacology: insights into therapeutic mechanisms. Pharmacological Reviews **70**:621–660.

Zarate CA, Brutsche N, Laje G, et al. (2012) Relationship of ketamine's plasma metabolites with response, diagnosis, and side effects in major depression. Biological Psychiatry **72**:331–338.

Zarate CA, Singh JB, Carlson PJ, et al. (2006) A randomized trial of an N-methyl-D-aspartate antagonist in treatment-resistant major depression. Archives of General Psychiatry **63**: 856–864.

CHAPTER 10

Risks and adverse events associated with the use of psychedelics

Joanna C. Neill, Mohammed Shahid, Rosalind Gittins, Anne K. Schlag, and Frank I. Tarazi

---

KEY POINTS

* Psychedelic medicine will provide much-needed treatment options for some mental health and neurological disorders in the near future.
* Certain gaps in knowledge exist that need to be addressed for improved treatment including:

  o full analysis of human receptor pharmacology;

  o further assessment of drug-drug interactions, particularly with antidepressant; antipsychotic and anticonvulsant medications.

  o Conducting clinical trials in ethnically diverse populations to better assess, benefits, risks, and adverse events of psychedelic agents in the society at large.

* Pharmacovigilance will be essential to ensure patient safety and tolerability to facilitate their wider use in clinical practice.

Introduction

As articulated throughout this book, psychedelic medicine represents a much-needed paradigm shift in the treatment of certain mental health disorders including treatment-resistant depression (TRD), post-traumatic stress disorders (PTSD), addictions and neurological disorders. This evolution is already well advanced, with an ever-increasing number of pharmaceutical and biotechnology companies working to develop new psychedelic molecules, formulations, and drug delivery systems (see detailed report from Psych Capital for status of the field as of October 2021: https://psych.global/report; and see Chapter 11). As access to these potent medicines is widened, so inevitably will the potential for adverse events in patients receiving them. The Drug Science team have investigated known risks, using currently available data from psychedelics used in clinical trials, in retreat settings and for recreation. Overall, we found low levels of adverse events, particularly of serious risks. This is in direct contrast with perceived risks, leading to undeserved stigmatization of psychedelics (Schlag et al.

2022). Furthermore, a recent trial in eighty-nine healthy participants showed that a single dose of 10 mg or 25 mg of psilocybin produced no serious adverse events (Rucker et al. 2022). Available evidence is however still limited and not always well documented in certain settings; furthermore, the number of clinical trials is small to date and generally not inclusive of a range of ethnicities and people with possible underlying health conditions. Thus, this chapter outlines the potential risks and adverse events associated with the classical psychedelics, as they are more likely to occur when access to psychedelic medicine is expanded into much larger and ethnically diverse patient populations for a broader range of indications. Specifically, we cover the pharmacology of serotonergic psychedelics, risks for adverse events and drug-drug interactions and make recommendations for postmarketing pharmacovigilance. These are all essential aspects to ensure that these medicines are safe and accessible for all appropriate patient groups. It should be noted that we do not cover MDMA or ketamine, as these are addressed in Chapters 4 and 9, respectively. Risks associated with ibogaine are detailed in Chapter 7. For specific risk issues related to the 'lesser-known' psychedelics such as muscimol, salvinorin A, mescaline, 2C-B, and 5-methoxy-DMT, the reader is referred to Chapter 8. Broader risks pertaining to the psychedelic field are considered in Chapter 11.

Risks for cardiovascular adverse reactions and other safety considerations

Serotonergic psychedelics cover a diverse set of molecules that have been categorized according to chemical class such as ergolines (e.g. D-lysergic acid diethylamide or LSD), tryptamines (e.g. the pro-drug psilocybin, N,N-dimethyltryptamine or DMT), and phenethylamines (e.g. mescaline). These agents bind to a broad range of central nervous system (CNS)-relevant receptors but share a common serotonergic pharmacology. Indeed, some groups such as the tryptamines show high homology with the core structure of the neurotransmitter 5-hydroxytryptamine (5-HT, serotonin). Because of their high affinity for 5-HT receptor subtypes, stimulation of these molecular targets, particularly the 5-HT2A receptor, seems to be the primary mode of action for their therapeutic effects (Nichols, 2016; Vollenweider & Preller, 2020) although involvement of other receptors (e.g. the 5-HT1A receptor) cannot be excluded (see also Chapter 11). Given that serotonergic psychedelics display strong structural similarity to 5-HT, it is not surprising that they show significant promiscuity across 5-HT receptor subtypes.

For a drug to meet the regulatory requirements for use in clinical practice, there must be a clear demonstration of effectiveness coupled with acceptable safety and tolerability profiles. The poly-pharmacology of serotonergic psychedelics may have implications for adverse events and safety risks. Therefore, we summarize current understanding of the human 5-HT receptor pharmacology of

LSD, psilocybin, psilocin (the active metabolite generated by de-phosphorylation of psilocybin), and DMT, and weigh implications for potential adverse events and safety risks. Gaps in knowledge are highlighted, alongside the need for the development and application of a translational pharmacokinetic and pharmacodynamic approach for full safety margin assessment.

Is there full clarity on clinically relevant human receptor pharmacology for serotonergic psychedelics?

Characterization of the human receptor pharmacology of the classic psychedelics has focused, to a large extent but not exclusively, on their effects on 5-HT receptor subtypes and associated impact on CNS neurotransmission and function. The 5-HT receptor superfamily consists of seven (5-HT1 to 5-HT7) subfamilies with a current total of nineteen receptor subtypes (see Barnes et al., 2020). With the exception of the 5-HT3 receptor, a ligand gated ion channel, all receptor subtypes belong to the class of G-protein coupled receptor (GPCR) characterized by a seven-transmembrane spanning segments. 5-HT plays an important neuromodulator role in the brain by influencing the function of other neurotransmitter pathways and impacting a variety of physiological processes such as sleep, mood, cognition, and appetite. In the periphery, serotonin acts like a hormone, influencing multiple organs including parts of the cardiovascular and gastrointestinal systems (Barnes et al., 2020).

Serotonergic psychedelics interact with a broad range of human 5-HT receptors with varying affinities and degree of agonism as well as subtle subtype selectivity (see Nichols, 2016). There is a general trend for them to show relatively higher affinity for the 5-HT2 receptor subfamily comprising of three receptor subtypes: 5-HT2A, 5-HT2B, and 5-HT2C. All three are present in brain tissue, with regional variation in expression pattern, which is likely to reflect differential physiological roles for each.

Pharmacological profiling of serotonergic psychedelics at human 5-HT2 receptor subtypes has currently focused on determining differing affinities as well as the potency in signal transduction based functional assays. Historically, this was conducted using animal tissue preparations and subsequently in cells expressing cloned rodent or human receptors. While considerable data has been generated, using varying methodologies and approaches, a systematic analysis of serotonergic psychedelics under appropriate uniform test conditions, is lacking. Table 10.1 summarizes human receptor pharmacology data for LSD, psilocybin, psilocin, and DMT (NIMH, PDSP https://pdsp.unc.edu/). It is clear that, despite the long history of these compounds, there are some important knowledge gaps. Since GPCR agonists preferentially bind to the high-affinity G-protein coupled state of the receptor, it is preferable to perform receptor binding analysis using an agonist radiolabelled ligand (e.g. ^{3}H-5HT). An antagonist radiolabelled ligand (e.g. ^{3}H-ketanserin) will be biased towards binding to the low-affinity site and may therefore yield a lower binding-affinity value for an agonist compound. Table

Table 10.1 Summary and comparison of the cloned human 5-HT2 receptor subtype binding-affinity values for 5-HT, d-LSD, psilocybin, psilocin, and DMT using agonist and antagonist radiolabelled ligand in addition to potency for receptor functional activity

Agonist (High-Affinity Site) Binding Assay (Ki nM)

Compound	5-HT2A	5-HT2B	5-HT2C	Reference
5-HT	16.2	13.5	5.8	Knight et al., 2004
	13.6	13.2	4.3	Song et al., 2005
	8.2	13	8.3	May et al., 2003
	9.1	ND	4.3	Janowsky et al., 2014
	7.77	9.46	15.5	Wainscott et al., 1996
d-LSD	0.76	0.98	1.10	Knight et al., 2004
	0.71	ND	2.91	Janowsky et al., 2014
	ND	3.7	ND	Wacker D et al., 2013
Psilocybin	NA	98.7	NA	PDSP Ki database
Psilocin	NA	NA	NA	PDSP Ki database
DMT	210	ND	166	Janowsky et al., 2014
	127	184	360	Keiser et al., 2009

Antagonist binding (Ki nM)

	5-HT2A	5-HT2B	5-HT2C	
5-HT	656, 341	2.81	18.2	PDSP Ki database
	12.6, 219		56.2	
	603, 63			
d-LSD	4.2	ND	15	Rickli et al., 2016
Psilocybin	10000	600	NA	PDSP
Psilocin	49	ND	94	Rickli A et al., 2016
	340	4.7	141	Ray, 2010
	107	4.6	97.3	Halberstadt, 2011
DMT	2323	108	335	Ray, 2010

Receptor functional activity
(calcium release[*] or phosphoinositide hydrolysis[†]: EC50 nM)

	5-HT2A EC50 Emax		5-HT2B EC50 Emax		5-HT2C EC50 Emax		
5-HT	30.9	102	2.08	106	5.75	97	Porter et al., 1999[*]
d-LSD	21.4	44	8.91	51	45.7	29	Porter et al., 1999[*]
	261	28	12000	71	ND		Rickli et al., 2016[*]
Psilocybin	3475	31	74	24	506	51	Sard et al., 2005[†]

Table 10.1 Continued							
Psilocin	24	43	58	45	30	51	Sard et al., 2005[†]
	45.2	76	ND		ND		Blough, et al., 2014[*]
	721	16	>20000		ND		Rickli et al., 2016[*]
DMT	76	40	3400	19	ND		Rickli et al., 2016[*]
	38.3	83	ND		ND		Blough et al.,2014[*]

Emax: % of maximum 5-HT response; ND: not determined; NA: not available.

Data sourced from: Blough BE. Interaction of psychoactive tryptamines with biogenic amine transporters and serotonin receptor subtypes. Psychopharmacology (Berl). 2014;231(21):4135–44; Halberstadt AL, Geyer MA. Multiple receptors contribute to the behavioral effects of indoleamine hallucinogens. Neuropharmacology. 2011; 61(3):364–81; Janowsky A, et al. Mefloquine and psychotomimetics share neurotransmitter receptor and transporter interactions in vitro. Psychopharmacology (Berl). 2014; 231(14):2771–83; Keiser MJ. Predicting new molecular targets for known drugs. Nature. 2009; 462(7270):175–81; Knight AR et al. Pharmacological characterisation of the agonist radioligand binding site of 5-HT(2A), 5-HT(2B) and 5-HT(2C) receptors. Naunyn Schmiedebergs Arch Pharmacol. 2004; 370(2):114–23; May JA, et al. A novel and selective 5-HT2 receptor agonist with ocular hypotensive activity: (S)-(+)-1-(2-aminopropyl)-8,9-dihydropyrano[3,2-e]indole. J Med Chem. 2003; 46(19):4188–95; Porter RH et al. Functional characterization of agonists at recombinant human 5-HT2A, 5-HT2B and 5-HT2C receptors in CHO-K1 cells. Br J Pharmacol. 1999; 128(1):13–20; Psychoactive Drug Screening Program (PDSP) K_i database; Ray TS. Psychedelics and the human receptorome. PLoS One. 2010; 2;5(2):e9019; Rickli A, et al. Receptor interaction profiles of novel psychoactive tryptamines compared with classic hallucinogens. Eur Neuropsychopharmacol. 2016; 26(8):1327–37; Sard H, et al. SAR of psilocybin analogs: discovery of a selective 5-HT 2C agonist. Bioorg Med Chem Lett. 2005; 15(20):4555–9; Song J, et al. Development of homogeneous high-affinity agonist binding assays for 5-HT2 receptor subtypes. Assay Drug Dev Technol. 2005; 3(6):649–659; Wainscott DB, et al. Pharmacologic characterization of the human 5-hydroxytryptamine2B receptor: evidence for species differences. J Pharmacol Exp Ther. 1996; 276(2):720–7.

10.1 shows that the binding affinity of 5-HT is lower when tested in an antagonist ligand binding assay. The same trend can be seen for LSD and DMT, but it is not clear if the same is true for psilocin, which appears not to have been tested using a radiolabelled ligand. This is an important scientific gap. Based on the antagonist binding assay, however, psilocin like LSD and DMT, binds to all three 5-HT2 receptor subtypes. Two published reports (see Table 10.1) indicate that psilocin has higher affinity, and therefore selectivity, for the 5-HT2B receptor when compared to 5-HT2A or 5-HT2C, but confirmation requires evaluation under more comparable assay conditions.

With regards to effects of LSD, psilocybin, psilocin, and DMT in cloned human 5-HT2 receptor functional assays, the overall data are rather sparse (Table 10.1). LSD is a partial agonist at 5-HT2A, 5-HT2B, and 5-HT2C receptors. Both psilocybin and psilocin show a similar profile to LSD. The effects of psilocybin may be, in part at least, due to generation of psilocin. However, Rickli and colleagues (2016) reported that psilocin had low potency in the 5-HT2B receptor assay (EC50 > 10uM). The reason for this discrepancy is not clear but may be related to differences in assay conditions and/or functional readout. DMT is also a partial agonist at 5-HT2A and 5-HT2B receptors, while no data for the 5-HT2C receptor has been reported.

Overall, the quality and completeness of the human receptor binding and functional assay data for LSD, psilocybin, psilocin, and DMT are limited and would benefit from a more systematic analysis at all three 5-HT2 receptor subtypes. A thorough receptor binding analysis and affinity determination is a key element in providing insight towards likely target engagement at doses used in clinical studies. Despite methodological variations and data heterogeneity, the available evidence does not support 5-HT2 subtype selectivity for LSD, psilocin, or DMT, suggesting that all three drugs are likely to engage all three 5-HT receptor subtypes. The relevance of differences in the degree of agonism is difficult to interpret given the nonphysiological nature of cloned cell lines and variation in methodology used by different research groups. Therefore, full clarity about the clinically relevant human receptor pharmacology of these agents remains to be established.

What are the main 5-HT2 receptor pharmacology based cardiovascular safety concerns for serotonergic psychedelics?

In addition to its neurotransmitter role in the brain, 5-HT acts like a hormone in other tissues, perhaps most importantly in the cardiovascular system (Machida et al., 2013; Rieder et al., 2021). It has been well documented that 5-HT modulates the function of vascular smooth muscle cells (VSMCs) and endothelial cells (ECs). Over 90% of 5-HT in the human body is generated by intestinal enterochromaffin cells; when released into the circulation, it is avidly taken up by platelets through the 5-HT transporter, allowing them to build a highly concentrated (around 0.4 mM) capacity (Flachaire et al., 1990). Platelet activation (e.g. because of vascular injury) provokes release of stored 5-HT, leading to an elevation in plasma 5-HT concentration which acts on VSMCs and ECs causing vasoconstriction and release of vasoactive mediators. Several members of the 5-HT receptor superfamily are believed to be expressed in the systemic vasculature, including the 5-HT2A receptor. This receptor is present on VSMCs and the VSMC contractile; thus, vasoconstriction effects of 5-HT are mainly mediated by stimulation of the 5-HT2A receptor, activation of which has also been implicated in the proliferation and migration of VSMCs (Matsusaka et al., 2005); this, together with other mediators, may have potential relevance for the pathogenesis of atherosclerosis (Rieder et al., 2021).

Given the primary 5-HT2A receptor pharmacology of serotonergic psychedelics, it is reasonable to expect some potential for cardiovascular adverse events through direct and/or indirect (sympathomimetic) mechanisms. Historical clinical experience with agents such as LSD (Passie et al., 2008; Dolder et al., 2017), psilocybin (Passie et al., 2002), and DMT (Carbonaro & Gatch, 2016), principally in healthy volunteers, highlights this as a potential issue, where relatively consistent (albeit transient) increases in heart rate and blood pressure have been observed. Given the mechanistic argument and observations in healthy volunteers, history of cardiovascular disease or anomalies have been general exclusion criteria for clinical trials.

LSD, psilocybin, psilocin, and DMT also show significant affinity for the 5-HT2B receptor. Although the data summarized in Table 10.1 have significant limitations, it is likely that psychedelic doses of these compounds will engage and modulate 5-HT2B receptor activity. How this may contribute towards their CNS related function is not clear; however, if these drugs are associated with 5-HT2B receptor stimulation, it does raise the need for checking potential liability regarding long-term cardiovascular and pulmonary safety.

The 5-HT2B receptor has been implicated in cardiac development and degenerative heart disease, as well as in drug-induced heart valve pathology (Hutcheson et al., 2011; Cavero & Guillon, 2014). These receptors are expressed in cardiac valve fibroblasts and are involved in maintaining normal structure but can also lead to damage following sustained overstimulation caused by disease (e.g. carcinoid tumours associated with a dramatic rise in plasma 5-HT) or drug toxicity. There are six well-known valvulopathic drugs: cabergoline, dihydroergotamine, ergonovine, methylergonovine, the fenfluramine metabolite norfenfluramine, and pergolide, whose toxic effects have been ascribed to their agonist activity at the human 5-HT2B receptor (see Table 10.2). Through Gq G-protein mediated coupling, 5-HT2B receptors stimulate phosphoinositide turnover, leading to activation of phospholipases C and A2. Subsequent elevation in intracellular calcium levels and downstream mitogenic action, through ERK1/2, Src, and protein kinase C (PKC) pathways leading to enhancement of TGF-β signalling, increases cellular proliferation promoting fibrosis and disruption of cardiac valve function. From a safety perspective, off-target 5HT2B agonist activity is considered as a 'red alert'. The general industry guide is to maintain at least a thirty- to one hundred–fold separation between on-target and off-target receptor affinities to provide an adequate safety margin during toxicological profiling (Cavero & Guillon, 2014). A more modest level of binding selectivity (approximately tenfold) over the off-target 5-HT2B receptor may also yield an adequate safety margin, as illustrated by the successful development of lorcaserin, a 5HT2C receptor selective agonist and anti-obesity agent (Thomsen et al., 2008). However, the approval of lorcaserin by the Food and Drug Administration (FDA) was conditional on additional long-term cardiovascular safety analysis, despite absence of a safety signal during preapproval trials (Cavero & Guillon, 2014). This highlights the importance that regulatory agencies attach to 5-HT2B receptor agonism as a significant safety alert, particularly for agents that will be used long-term. Consequently, barring any compelling argument based around risk-benefit analysis, most pharmaceutical and biotechnology companies try to avoid investing in developing drugs known to have significant off-target 5-HT2B agonism liability.

As detailed in Chapter 3, long-term use is not the intended mode of treatment for serotonergic psychedelics such as psilocybin, and this has implications for the 5-HT2B receptor agonism related risk-benefit analysis. Based on recent studies in TRD, PTSD, and anxiety, it seems that up to three doses, given under supervision

Table 10.2 Summary of the human 5-HT2B receptor binding and signalling pathway activation data for 5-HT, DOI, d-LSD, psilocybin, psilocin and six drugs known to cause cardiac valve damage along with their free maximum concentration in plasma at clinically used doses

Compound	Receptor Binding Ki	Phosphoinositide Metabolism EC50	%Emax	Calcium Release EC50	%Emax	Arrestin Translocation EC50	%Emax	ERK2 Phosphorylation EC50	%Emax	Transcription Factor Activity EC50	%Emax	Free Plasma Cmax
5-HT	13.5	10.7	100	1.78	100	16.6	100	0.37	100	0.72	100	–
DOI	43.7	64.6	103	1.44	88.2	102	96	5.50	54	13.8	107	–
d-LSD	0.98 3.7	?		8.91 12000	51 71	?		?		?		?
Psilocybin	98.7	74	24	?		?		?		?		?
Psilocin	4.7	58	45	>20000		?		?		?		?
DMT	184	?		3400	19	?		?		?		?
Heart valve toxic drugs												
Cabergoline	1.2-1.3	6.6	7	398	98.5	5.89	90.6	3.63	60.1	0.79	108	1.59
Dihydroergotamine	152	33.1	76	5012	81.6	22.4	175	5.37	70.6	4.78	92	0.35-0.53
Ergonovine	1.4	2.29	22.2	70.8	39.7	15.1	74.7	3.31	57	0.93	54.3	3.56
Methylergonovine	0.5	3.01	18.7	21.4	49.5	1.10	102	1.66	52.5	0.50	56	12
Norfenfluramine	100	186	84	2.45	107	129	52	1.41	75	15.5	101	44;77
Pergolide	7.1;14	115	95	74.1	88.5	18.6	92	1.02	79	19.1	108	100:0.87

Ki, EC50, and plasma Cmax values in nM; %Emax: is % of maximum 5-HT response.

Data sourced and adapted from: Cavero I, Guillon JM. Safety Pharmacology assessment of drugs with biased 5-HT(2B) receptor agonism mediating cardiac valvulopathy. J Pharmacol Toxicol Methods. 2014; 69(2):150–61; Knight AR et al. Pharmacological characterisation of the agonist radioligand binding site of 5-HT(2A), 5-HT(2B) and 5-HT(2C) receptors. Naunyn Schmiedebergs Arch Pharmacol. 2004; 370(2):114–23; Papoian T, et al. Regulatory Forum Review*: utility of in vitro secondary pharmacology data to assess risk of drug-induced valvular heart disease in humans: regulatory considerations. Toxicol Pathol. 2017; 45(3):381–388; Huang XP, Setola V, Yadav PN, Allen JA, Rogan SC, Hanson BJ, Revankar C, Robers M, Doucette C, Roth BL. Parallel functional activity profiling reveals valvulopathogens are potent 5-hydroxytryptamine(2B) receptor agonists: implications for drug safety assessment. Mol Pharmacol. 2009; 76(4):710–22.

at weekly (or longer) intervals and with psychological support, has an enduring effect, obviating the need for daily administration. Nevertheless, the potential safety risk should be evaluated using regulatory advice. Papoian et al. (2017) have provided some considerations in this respect, based on a correlational analysis examining human 5-HT2B receptor affinity or potency in a variety of functional assays relative to exposure unbound drug plasma Cmax for several known drugs associated with heart valve damage. They suggested that safety multiples based on Ki values may be a better predictor than potency values from functional assays. Potency and activity in functional assays based on heterologous cloned cell lines should be interpreted with caution as they can be affected by nonphysiological receptor overexpression. High receptor expression density, for example, can lead to promiscuous G-protein coupling or differential activity across multiple signalling pathways, as well as risk of constitutive receptor activity. It has also been suggested that using multiple functional readouts may confer some value in identifying the most-sensitive signalling pathway as well as opportunity for pattern-based analysis (Huang et al., 2009). This is exemplified by the data summarized in Table 10.2 for known valvopathic drugs, which generally show a higher potency in a transcription factor assay compared to other signalling assays. Such detailed functional analysis has not been reported for LSD, psilocybin, psilocin, or DMT, and it would be informative to learn how these molecules differ in their signalling signature from drugs known to cause heart valve toxicity.

In summary, it is clear that there are gaps in knowledge of the human receptor pharmacology of LSD, psilocin, and DMT, and these need to be comprehensively addressed. The pharmacological strategy adopted by Shahid and colleagues (2009) for the characterization of the atypical antipsychotic drug asenapine may be useful to consider in this respect. Application of an appropriately designed translational pharmacodynamic or pharmacokinetic approach is required to provide a better insight into which receptors are being engaged at therapeutic doses.

Drug-drug interactions with psychotropic drugs

Antidepressant medicines

Results from recent small-scale clinical trials have provided robust evidence for the beneficial therapeutic effects of many of the psychedelics described in this book, notably for hard-to-treat psychiatric disorders including TRD and PTSD. TRD and PTSD patients are commonly treated with several classes of antidepressant medicines such as selective serotonin reuptake inhibitors (SSRIs) and serotonin and noradrenaline reuptake inhibitors (SNRIs). These medicines potentiate serotonergic neurotransmission by blocking the reuptake of 5-HT into presynaptic vesicles (Feighner, 1999). On the other hand, direct action at the 5-HT2A receptor appears to mediate the neurobiological effects of psychedelics as described above. As wider patient access is enabled, it is increasingly likely that TRD and PTSD patients will be treated with psychedelics as adjunctive therapy to their existing antidepressants, including SSRIs and SNRIs. However, several studies have highlighted the possible risks and adverse events that may result from the interactions between antidepressants and psychedelics. These studies have raised concerns that combining SSRIs or SNRIs with psychedelics may augment 5-HT neurotransmission, trigger serotonin syndrome, or blunt the subjective effects of psychedelics.

Serotonin syndrome

Serotonin (5-HT) syndrome is a potentially lethal adverse drug reaction most likely to occur as a result of overstimulation of 5-HT neurotransmission owing to one or more 5-HT-stimulating drugs, with increasing risk at higher doses (Boyer & Shannon, 2005). The severity of 5-HT syndrome can vary from mild to life-threatening. Symptoms typically include tremor or loss of muscle coordination, tachycardia, hypertension, dilated pupils, and agitation. In severe 5-HT syndrome, several life-threatening signs can be observed, including high fever, seizures, delirium, heart arrhythmia, and loss of consciousness (Mills, 1997; Birmes et al., 2003). The pathophysiology of 5-HT syndrome is not well defined, though it is believed that stimulation of 5-HT2A receptors and to a lesser extent, 5-HT1A receptors contribute significantly (Francescangeli et al., 2019). Increases in other neurotransmitter levels including dopamine and noradrenaline have also been linked to increases in 5-HT levels and worsening of clinical outcomes (Mills, 1997; Brimes et al., 2003).

In addition, several psychedelics, such as LSD and 5-Meo-DMT, are metabolized by CYP2D6, a member of the cytochrome P450 family of enzymes involved in the oxidative metabolism (Shen et al., 2010; Luethi et al., 2019). A number of SSRIs are potent inhibitors of CYP2D6 (Hiemke & Härtter, 2000), hence coadministration of SSRIs with psychedelics may reduce the levels of CYP2D6 available to metabolize psychedelics, which will elevate levels and further increase 5-HT neurotransmission and the risk of serotonin syndrome. Polymorphic variations in the CYP2D6 gene and their differential metabolic activities have also been suggested to contribute to serotonin syndrome (Kaneda et al., 2002).

These observations have led to recommendations to slowly taper then stop treatments with antidepressants for at least several weeks prior to the initiation of psychedelic therapy, to prevent reduction of treatment response to psychedelic-assisted psychotherapy (Feduccia et al., 2021) and reduce the risk of 5-HT syndrome (Malcolm & Thomas, 2021). Nonetheless, patients who were previously treated with different classes of antidepressants and switched to receive psychedelic therapy should be monitored closely for early signs of 5-HT syndrome.

Reduction of subjective effects of psychedelics

Clinical evidence suggests that chronic use of SSRIs, tricyclic antidepressants (TCAs), and monoamine oxidase inhibitors (MAOIs) diminishes the subjective effects of psychedelics (Bonson & Murphy, 1995; Bonson et al., 1996). The mechanisms behind this effect remain to be fully clarified, but SSRI-induced downregulation of 5-HT2A receptors, as well as MAOI-induced 5-HT2A receptor desensitization, presumably contribute to this phenomenon (Johnson et al., 2008). This reduction may lead to people increasing the dose of psychedelics to achieve the required subjective effects, which will substantially increase the risk of 5-HT syndrome and other serious adverse events. Moreover, SSRIs have been shown to potentiate the emergence of LSD-induced flashbacks even months after stopping LSD use (Markel et al., 1994). It remains to be determined whether this can occur with other psychedelics.

Psilocybin and antidepressant medicines

Two recent trials examined the interaction between the psychedelic psilocybin and antidepressants. The first trial investigated the response to two treatment sessions of psilocybin (25 mg), separated by sixteen days, in twenty-three healthy participants (twelve men and eleven women) after pretreatment with the antidepressant escitalopram or placebo. Pretreatment consisted of 10 mg escitalopram daily for seven days, followed by 20 mg daily for seven days, including the day of psilocybin administration, or fourteen days of placebo pretreatment before psilocybin administration. Escitalopram pretreatment did not reduce the positive mood effects of psilocybin and furthermore significantly reduced anxiety, cardiovascular side effects, and other adverse effects, compared with placebo pretreatment. In addition, escitalopram did not alter 5-HT2A receptor gene expression before psilocybin administration, prolong QTc intervals, or increase circulating brain-derived neurotrophic factor (BDNF) levels before or after psilocybin administration (Becker et al., 2021). These preliminary results suggest that escitalopram may even enhance the tolerability of psilocybin, but it is not clear whether this can be extrapolated to people with clinical depression treated with SSRIs long-term.

A recent open-label clinical study examined the effects of concomitant SSRI therapy with psilocybin (25 mg) in nineteen TRD patients. The trial reported similar clinical outcomes to another randomized double-blind trial which evaluated the effects of psilocybin in TRD patients after being withdrawn from their SSRIs. In addition, psilocybin was generally well-tolerated, and there were no life-threatening adverse events or other side effects leading to disabilities or hospitalization, and no increased risk of suicidal ideation or behaviour or intentional self-injury (Compass Pathways Press Release, 2021). This trial result awaits peer review, but together these studies argue against warnings of combining psilocybin with SSRIs. However, larger trials are required that investigate the interaction of psilocybin and other psychedelics with other SSRIs and other antidepressants, including full investigation of pharmacokinetic interactions.

Anticonvulsant and antipsychotic medicines

The interactions between psychedelics and anticonvulsant and antipsychotic drugs are less well documented than interactions with antidepressants. However, the available studies reported potentially significant interactions. For example, analysis of reports revealed that coadministration of psychedelics with lithium, but not lamotrigine, increased the risks of seizure and dissociative effects in bipolar disorder patients (Nayak et al., 2021). Antipsychotic-induced blockade and down regulation of the 5-HT2A receptor may blunt the subjective effects of psychedelics, and subsequently increase the risk of 5-HT syndrome (Howland, 2016). Additional clinical studies are still required to better characterize these interactions and their clinical impact.

Postmarketing pharmacovigilance of psychedelic medicines

Pharmacovigilance continues once medicinal products are approved and marketed. When used in clinical practice, patients receiving medication and the setting in which they are used are not controlled in the same way as during premarketing clinical trials. This means that a more diverse population with a wider range of characteristics and comorbidities will access the novel therapy, supporting the need for careful monitoring. The coadministration of other medicines which can give rise to drug-drug interactions are also more likely to feature (see above).

Drug developers are required to submit their proactive risk planning measures to regulators, outlining how they intend to monitor and mitigate risks following product approval. This is informed by the theoretical mechanism of the medicines' known pharmacodynamics, associated pharmacokinetics, and the condition it is to be used for, in addition to what has already been established in premarketing studies. Furthermore, to support ongoing regulatory decision-making, postauthorization safety studies are conducted to review postmarketing safety data and establish the effectiveness of the risk-management measures.

Postmarketing requirements are determined by regulatory authorities such as the European Medicines Agency (EMA) and the United States FDA. In the European market, medicines that are subject to monitoring that is more intense are labelled with a black triangle, which usually remains in situ for five years (BNF, 2021). In the UK, the Yellow Card reporting scheme is operated by the Medicines and Healthcare Regulatory Agency (MHRA, 2021). It relies on the voluntary reporting of adverse events (and other issues) by patients and healthcare professionals, with the aim of providing an early warning system. This system incorporates reports associated with black triangle medicines, and equivalent systems operate in other countries. For example, in 2021, the FDA launched a publicly accessible dashboard for drugs where there are particular safety concerns and can introduce additional measures such as certification of healthcare professionals or dispensaries, define patient monitoring requirements, or require their enrolment in registries via the Risk Evaluation and Mitigation Strategy (REMS) program. Contemporaneous reporting of concerns is important to ensure that any issues are readily identified and reviewed. This enables regulators to monitor for trends and continuously ensure that the perceived therapeutic benefits associated with the product's use outweigh the potential negative consequences. If adverse events arise, additional warnings may be issued; the way in which the product can be used may be subject to further restrictions; or on rare occasions, withdrawal of the product from the market may also occur. An example of this is thalidomide, which was used for morning sickness and resulted in birth defects, and was withdrawn in the 1960s, but has since been reintroduced and successfully used within patient safety programmes for conditions such as leprosy and multiple myeloma (Vargesson & Stephens, 2021).

The psychedelics currently used in clinical trials are not newly produced compounds; indeed, there is a notable amount of information relating to their recreational use, certainly more than with new chemical entities (Schlag et al., 2022). However, there remains a paucity of recently published evidence to support their use in clinical practice in accordance with the level of rigour currently required by regulators. This highlights the importance of ongoing research and any consequent marketing authorization with associated pharmacovigilance requirements. Additionally, psychedelics are highly controlled drugs, making their use subject to additional scrutiny. Unfortunately, their Schedule 1 status makes research challenging to conduct because of the associated increased costs and logistics needed to meet the requirements of controlled drug legislation (Nutt et al., 2020; Rucker, 2015; see Howard et al., 2021 for an in-depth qualitative analysis of the barriers faced by Schedule 1 researchers in the UK).

Because of the risks associated with controlled drugs, such as diversion, their use is subject to additional monitoring. Sharing of intelligence, identifying concerns, learning from incidents, and highlighting issues in relation to specific products, patients, or healthcare professionals across care systems are important so that prompt action can be taken to mitigate risks. Following the Shipman Inquiry, additional UK controlled drug regulations were introduced (National Archives, 2013), requiring designated bodies such as NHS Trusts to appoint Accountable Officers for controlled drugs. Controlled Drug Local Intelligence Networks provide a framework for reporting measures. Any issues with medical psychedelics would also be covered, and should any issues arise, particularly in relation to suspected diversion, established systems should enable prompt detection.

Conclusions

The research into psychedelic medicine presented here reveals a need for comprehensive analysis of the human receptor pharmacology, to inform risk-benefit analysis at clinical doses. Available evidence suggests that interaction of psilocybin with current antidepressant medication may be minimal, although further work is needed with larger trials and other psychedelics. Pharmacovigilance is likely to be as critical for patient safety as with a new chemical entity, in spite of the use of psychedelics for spiritual and recreational purposes for many years. Much work remains to be done to enable safe patient access as the field continues to build on the positive and highly encouraging results from the clinical trials conducted to date. This includes increases in patient diversity in trials, extensive analysis of the pharmacology including human receptor selectivity analysis of the various compounds, and further and larger studies investigating drug-drug interactions, particularly with anticonvulsants and antipsychotics. This is one of the most important and exciting innovations in psychiatry for over half a century. In order to maximize the potential for patient benefit, it is essential that we proceed carefully and conduct all essential safety and risk-benefit evaluation at each stage.

Disclosures

JCN is a scientific adviser to Beckley Psytech, Octarine Bio and Albert Labs. AKS is scientific adviser to PsychCapital and is Head of Research of Drug Science. Drug Science receives an unrestricted educational grant from a consortium of medical psychedelics companies to further its mission, that is the pursuit of an unbiased and scientific assessment of drugs regardless of their regulatory class. JCN and RG are expert committee members of Drug Science. JCN chairs the Drug Science Medical Psychedelics Working Group. All Drug Science committee members (including the chair) are unpaid by Drug Science for their effort and commitment to this organization. MS and FIT report no conflict of interest. None of the authors would benefit from the wider prescribing of medical psychedelics in any form.

REFERENCES

Barnes NM, Ahern GP, Becamel C, et al. (2020) International Union of Basic and Clinical Pharmacology. CX. Classification of receptors for 5-hydroxytryptamine: pharmacology and function. Pharmacology Reviews 73:310–520.

Becker AM, Holze F, Grandientti T, et al. (2021) Acute effects of psilocybin after escitalopram or placebo pretreatment in a randomized, double-blind, placebo-controlled, crossover study in healthy subjects. Clinical Pharmacology and Therapeutics doi:10.1002/cpt.2487.

Becker AM, Holze F, Grandinetti T, et al. (2022) Acute Effects of Psilocybin After Escitalopram or Placebo Pretreatment in a Randomized, Double-Blind, Placebo-Controlled, Crossover Study in Healthy Subjects. Clin Pharmacol Ther. Apr;111(4): 886–895. doi: 10.1002/cpt.2487.

Birmes P, Coppin D, Schmitt L, Lauque D (2003) Serotonin syndrome: a brief review. CMAJ 168:1439–1442.

Bonson K, Buckholtz JW, Murphy DL (1996) Chronic administration of serotonergic antidepressants attenuates the subjective effects of LSD in humans. Neuropsychopharmacology 14:425–436.

Bonson KR, Murphy DL (1995) Alterations in responses to LSD in humans associated with chronic administration of tricyclic antidepressants, monoamine oxidase inhibitors or lithium. Behavioural Brain Research 73:229–233.

Boyer EW, Shannon M (2005) The serotonin syndrome. New England Journal of Medicine 352:1112–11120.

British National Formulary (BNF) (2021) Adverse reactions to drugs. https://bnf.nice.org.uk/guidance/adverse-reactions-to-drugs.html.

Carbonaro TM, Gatch MB (2016) Neuropharmacology of N,N-dimethyltryptamine. Brain Research Bulletin **126**(Pt 1):74–88.

Cavero I, Guillon JM (2014) Safety pharmacology assessment of drugs with biased 5-HT(2B) receptor agonism mediating cardiac valvulopathy. Journal of Pharmacological and Toxicological Methods **69**:150–161.

COMPASS Pathways (2021) Press Release: COMPASS Pathways announces positive outcome of 25mg COMP360 psilocybin therapy as adjunctive to SSRI antidepressants in open-label treatment resistant depression study. December 13, 2021.

Dolder PC, Schmid Y, Steuer AE, et al. (2017) Pharmacokinetics and pharmacodynamics of lysergic acid diethylamide in healthy subjects. Clinical Pharmacokinetics **56**:1219–1230.

Feduccia AA, Jerome L, Mithoefer MC, Holland J (2021) Discontinuation of medications classified as reuptake inhibitors affects treatment response of MDMA-assisted psychotherapy. Psychopharmacology **238**:581–588.

Feighner JP (1999) Mechanism of action of antidepressant medications. Journal of Clinical Psychiatry **60**(Suppl 4):4–11.

Flachaire E, Beney C, Berthier A, et al. (1990) Determination of reference values for serotonin concentration in platelets of healthy newborns, children, adults, and elderly subjects by HPLC with electrochemical detection. Clinical Chemistry **36**:2117–2120.

Francescangeli J, Karamchandani K, Powell M, Bonavia A (2019) The serotonin syndrome: from molecular mechanisms to clinical practice. International Journal of Molecular Sciences **20**:2288.

Goodwin GM, Aaronson ST, Alvarez O, et al. (2022) Single-dose psilocybin for a treatment-resistant episode of major depression. The New England Journal of Medicine **387**:1637–1648.

Hiemke C, Härtter S (2000) Pharmacokinetics of selective serotonin reuptake inhibitors. Pharmacology and Therapeutics **85**:11–28.

Howard A, Neill JC, Schlag AK, Lennox C (2021) Schedule 1 barriers to research in the UK: an in-depth qualitative analysis. Drug Science Policy and Law **7**:1–13.

Howland RH (2016) Antidepressant, antipsychotic, and hallucinogen drugs for the treatment of psychiatric disorders: a convergence at the serotonin-2A receptor. Journal of Psychosocial Nursing and Mental Health Services **54**:21–24.

Huang XP, Setola V, Yadav PN, et al. (2009) Parallel functional activity profiling reveals valvulopathogens are potent 5-hydroxytryptamine(2B) receptor agonists: implications for drug safety assessment. Molecular Pharmacology **76**:710–22.

Hutcheson JD, Setola V, Roth BL, Merryman WD (2011) Serotonin receptors and heart valve disease—it was meant 2B. Pharmacology and Therapeutics **132**:146–157.

Johnson MW, Richards WA, Griffiths RR (2008) Human hallucinogen research: guidelines for safety. Journal of Psychopharmacology **22**:603–620.

Kaneda Y, Kawamura I, Fujii A, Ohmori T (2002) Serotonin syndrome: 'potential' role of the CYP2D6 genetic polymorphism in Asians. International Journal of Neuropsychopharmacology **5**:105–106.

Luethi D, Hoener MC, Krähenbühl S, et al. (2019) Cytochrome P450 enzymes contribute to the metabolism of LSD to nor-LSD and 2-oxo-3-hydroxy-LSD: implications for clinical LSD use. Biochemical Pharmacology 164:129–138.

Machida T, Iizuka K, Hirafuji M (2013) 5-hydroxytryptamine and its receptors in systemic vascular walls. Biological and Pharmaceutical Bulletin 36:1416–1419.

Malcolm B, Thomas K (2021) Serotonin toxicity of serotonergic psychedelics. Psychopharmacology doi:10.1007/s00213-021-05876-x.

Malcolm B, Thomas K. (2022) Serotonin toxicity of serotonergic psychedelics. Psychopharmacology (Berl). Jun;239(6):1881–1891. doi: 10.1007/s00213-021-05876-x.

Markel H, Lee A, Homes RD, Domino EF (1994) LSD flashback syndrome exacerbated by selective serotonin reuptake inhibitor antidepressants in adolescents. Journal of Pediatrics 125(5 Pt 1):817–819.

Matsusaka S, Wakabayashi I (2005) 5-Hydroxytryptamine augments migration of human aortic smooth muscle cells through activation of RhoA and ERK. Biochemical and Biophysical Research Communications 337:916–21.

Medicines and Healthcare Regulatory Agency (MHRA) (2021) Yellow Card. https://yellowcard.mhra.gov.uk/.

Mills KC (1997) Serotonin syndrome: a clinical update. Critical Care Clinics 13:763–783.

National Archives (2013) Controlled drugs (supervision of management and use) regulations. https://www.legislation.gov.uk/uksi/2013/373/contents/made.

Nayak SM, Gukasyan N, Barrett FS, et al. (2021) Classic psychedelic coadministration with lithium, but not lamotrigine, is associated with seizures: an analysis of online psychedelic experience reports. Pharmacopsychiatry 54:240–245.

Nichols DE (2016) Psychedelics. Pharmacology Reviews 68:264–355.

Nutt DJ, Erritzoe D, Carhart-Harris R (2020) Psychedelic psychiatry's brave new world. Cell Press.

Papoian T, Jagadeesh G, Saulnier M, et al. (2017) Regulatory forum review: utility of in vitro secondary pharmacology data to assess risk of drug-induced valvular heart disease in humans—regulatory considerations. Toxicologic Pathology 45:381–388.

Passie T, Halpern JH, Stichtenoth DO, et al. (2008) The pharmacology of lysergic acid diethylamide: a review. CNS Neuroscience Therapeutics 14:295–314.

Passie T, Seifert J, Schneider U, Emrich HM (2002) The pharmacology of psilocybin. Addiction Biology 7:357–364.

Rieder M, Gauchel N, Bode C, Duerschmied D (2021) Serotonin: a platelet hormone modulating cardiovascular disease. Journal of Thrombosis and Thrombolysis 52:42–47.

Rucker J (2015) Psychedelic drugs should be legally reclassified so that researchers can investigate their therapeutic potential. BMJ 350:h2902.

Rucker J, Marwood L, Ajantaival R-LJ, et al. (2022) The effects of psilocybin on cognitive and emotional functions in healthy participants: Results from a phase 1, randomised, placebo-controlled trial involving simultaneous psilocybin administration and preparation. Journal of Psychopharmacology 36:114–125. doi:10.1177/02698811211064720.

Schlag AK, Aday J, Salam I, et al. (2022) Adverse effects of psychedelics: From anecdotes and misinformation to systematic science. J Psychopharmacol. 36(3):258–272. doi: 10.1177/02698811211069100.

Shahid M, Walker GB, Zorn SH, Wong EH (2009) Asenapine: a novel psychopharmacologic agent with a unique human receptor signature. Journal of Psychopharmacology 23:65–73.

Shen H-W, Jiang X-L, Winter JC, Yu A-M (2010) Psychedelic 5-methoxy-N,N-dimethyltryptamine: metabolism, pharmacokinetics, drug interactions, and pharmacological actions. Current Drug Metabolism 11:659–666.

Thomsen WJ, Grottick AJ, Menzaghi F, et al. (2008) Lorcaserin, a novel selective human 5-hydroxytryptamine2C agonist: in vitro and in vivo pharmacological characterization. Journal of Pharmacology and Experimental Therapeutics 325:577–587.

Vargesson N, Stephens T (2021) Thalidomide: history, withdrawal, renaissance, and safety concerns. Expert Opin Drug Saf. 20(12):1455–1457. doi: 10.1080/14740338.2021.1991307.

Vollenweider FX, Preller KH (2020) Psychedelic drugs: neurobiology and potential for treatment of psychiatric disorders. Nature Reviews Neuroscience 21:611–624.

Wang RZ, Vashistha V, Kaur S, Houchens NW (2016) Serotonin syndrome: preventing, recognizing and treating it. Cleveland Clinical Journal of Medicine 83:810–817.

CHAPTER 11

Psychedelics as psychiatric medicines: Current challenges and future prospects

David Castle, Nicole Ledwos, and David Nutt

KEY POINTS

- There has been a massive resurgence of interest in psychedelic and 'psychedelic-like' drugs for mental health and addiction, over the last decade.
- Understanding the mechanisms of action of these disparate compounds can inform further treatment development.
- Despite exciting outcomes from clinical trials, most remain small-scale and require replication.
- Long-term efficacy and safety need to be determined.
- It is important for clinicians and regulators to determine the best way in which psychedelic-assisted psychotherapy can be integrated into care pathways and made accessible to those in most need.

It is clear from contributions to this book that the psychedelic renaissance is here. Tracking longitudinal trends in scientific publications attests to the sheer number of scientists around the world who have turned their attention to the field (see Figure 11.1). The National Institutes for Health in the United States held a two-day online forum in January 2022 on the topic and attracted over 4,000 participants. And the number of registered clinical trials is multiplying dramatically (Figure 11.2).

Understanding this burgeoning field requires contextualization. First, the field is very much overdue in terms of medications for maladies of the mind with truly novel mechanisms of action. The ability of modern science to unveil neurobiological underpinnings of such mechanisms (e.g. functional MRI, MRS, and PET) lends scientific 'credibility' and reassures many that there is true 'science' behind the hype. Indeed the first UK trial of psilocybin for depression (Carhart-Harris et al., 2016) developed from the finding that, in healthy volunteers, it attenuated activity in brain regions that were known to be overactive in depression—a powerful example of translational medicine (Nutt, 2020). Second, there is a mystical allure that accompanies the psychedelics and an association with notions such as Huxley's 'Doors of Perception', the 1960s culture of freedom and

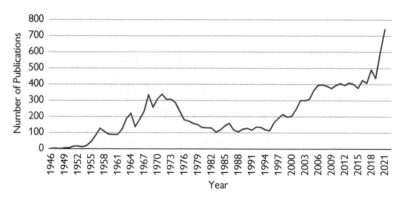

Figure 11.1 PubMed psychedelic publications per year. The chart includes all psychedelic substances mentioned in this book.

experimentation, and the longstanding use in the context of religious ceremonies dating back centuries and reaching across cultures (see Chapter 1). Third, the fact that this paradigm embraces both a biological and a psychological component to therapy allows a challenge to the reductionism and retreat into 'camps' associated with the moves (in North America most markedly) away from psychodynamic

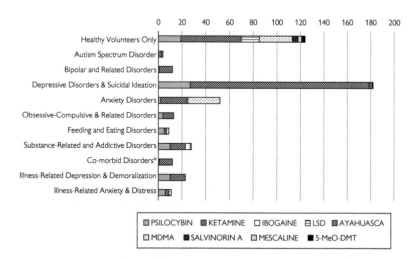

Figure 11.2 Registered clinical trials for psychedelic compounds. *Comorbid disorders include depression and alcohol use disorder, posttraumatic stress disorder and depression, posttraumatic stress disorder and chronic pain, and depression and opioid-use disorder.

psychotherapy towards neurobiology, from the 1990s. Fourth, is the recognition that mental health and addiction problems are increasing and exacerbated markedly in the context of the COVID-19 pandemic and its sequelae. And finally, inevitably, is the potential for large amounts of money to be made: Phelps et al. (2022) reported in January 2022 that there were already fifty publicly traded companies with an interest in 'psychedelic-like' drugs, and that projections for market growth were from a base of $2bn in 2022 to $10.7bn by 2027.

However, there is so much more to learn and to understand about this field, and there are also a number of potential pitfalls and dangers that bear consideration. This chapter outlines these sets of issues, and paints a picture as to how the immediate future might look for this emerging paradigm.

The need for more rigorous large-scale randomized controlled trials

Despite the fact that most modern trials of psychedelics and related agents follow more rigorous methodology than those employed in the 'first-wave' studies in the 1950s and 1960s (see Chapter 1), the overall evidence base of these more recent studies is actually quite small. Probably most compelling in terms of large-scale randomized controlled trials (RCTs) are those using ketamine to target depression (Chapter 10). Intravenous administration is associated with rapid antidepressant and antisuicidal effects, but the intravenous route has obvious logistical problems associated with it. In terms of oral dosing, Rosenblat et al. (2019) reviewed thirteen clinical trials of oral ketamine for depression (including two RCTs, both of which were considered at high risk of bias) and found effects on mood were not as rapid as for intravenous administration. Searching for an alternative mode of delivery, the s-enantiomer of ketamine has been developed as an intranasal formulation, which has been approved in a number of countries as an add-on treatment for depression resistant to SSRIs and related antidepressants (TRD) (Kaur et al., 2021). Exploring different formulations, delivery methods, dosing, and target symptoms will require further large-scale RCTs. In addition, RCT protocols need to be expanded to address the longevity of treatment effects and the rates of relapse over long periods of time.

MDMA has the strongest support for the treatment of posttraumatic stress disorder (PTSD), across a number of phase 2 studies (Chapter 4). These findings have recently been supported by a large-scale, multicentre, placebo-controlled phase 3 RCT of ninety participants with PTSD (Mitchell et al., 2021). There were high statistically significant advantages for MDMA vs. placebo, on the Clinician-Administered PTSD scale for DSM-5 (CAPS-5) ($p < 0.0001$; $d = 0.91$) as well as the Sheehan Disability Scale. Such large-scale, multicentre studies, with mechanisms to ensure treatment fidelity across sites, to optimize blinding (e.g. using a centralized pool of rating personnel who never assess the same participant more than once) and with adequate statistical power, need to be emulated for the classical psychedelics and emerging other related agents to establish efficacy and safety.

Psilocybin has the next most evidence, notably for end-of-life existential depression and anxiety in people with cancer (Chapter 3). A recent meta-analysis of four studies (n = 117) reported a pre-post effect size (Hedges' g) for anxiety of 1.38 (95%CI 0.78–1.99) and for depression of 1.47 (95%CI 0.72–2.21) (Goldberg et al., 2020). Psilocybin was well tolerated across all these studies, and benefits largely endured at follow-up. In contrast, the evidence for efficacy for psilocybin for major depression is relatively small. The seminal TRD study of Carhart-Harris et al. (2016) was an open trial with only twelve participants, albeit it achieved a large effect size for efficacy on depression rated by the QIDS-SR16 (Hedges' g 3.1 (95%CI 9.15–14.35; p = 0.002) at week one of follow-up, and 2.0 (95%CI 5.69–12.71; p = 0.003) at three months). Davis et al. (2021) randomly assigned people with major depressive disorder to two psilocybin sessions (20 mg/70 kg and 30 mg/70 kg) (n = 15) or waitlist (n = 12), and reported rapid benefits for PAP, with effect sizes (Cohen d) at five weeks of 2.5 (95%CI 1.4–3.5; p < 0.001) and 2.6 (95%CI 1.5–3.7; p < 0.001) at eight weeks. Finally, Goodwin et al. (2022) compared 10 mg (n = 75) and 25 mg (n = 79) doses of psilocybin with 1 mg (n = 79: considered a placebo dose) in a double-blind controlled trial of patients with treatment-resistant depression. Depression scores on the MADRS (least-squares mean changes) were −12.0 for 25 mg (difference from 1mg group −6.6 (95% CI − 10.2–−2.9; p < 0.001)); −7.9 for 10 mg (difference from 1mg group −2.5 (95%CI − 6.2-1.2; p = 0.18); and −5.4 for 1 mg. There was a relatively high rate of reported adverse events (179 of 233 participants (77%)), including headache, nausea, and dizziness. Suicidality was also observed in patients across all dose groups.

There are very few head-to-head trials comparing PAP and another active compound, whilst controlling for the psychotherapeutic component of the intervention. The stand-out exception is the comparator trial of psilocybin and escitalopram, conducted by Carhart-Harris et al. (2021). This trial was also relatively small (total n = 59) and showed similar reductions on the QIDS-SR (16 at six weeks (−8.0 +/ −1.0 points for psilocybin and −6.0 +/ −1.0 for escitalopram); p = 0.17). However, response and remission rates favoured psilocybin (response 70% vs. 48%: difference 22%; 95%CI −3–48; remission 57% vs. 28%; difference 28%; 95%CI 2–54). Other outcomes were generally better for the psilocybin group (not corrected for multiple comparisons); adverse events were largely equal. Turning to alcohol use disorder, Bogenschutz et al. (2022) saw a significant reduction in heavy drinking days with psilocybin vs. diphenhydramine in ninety-three patients, over thirty-two weeks of follow-up (standard mean difference 13.9% (95%CI 3.0–24.7)). Further placebo-controlled and head-to-head studies across depression, alcohol use disorder, and potentially other psychiatric disorders are warranted, albeit the issue of comparator choice, as well as blinding, remain challenges (see below). Optimal dosing is also debateable, with evidence of an inverted U effect and a suggested 'sweet spot' at 30–35 mg/70 kg, for psilocybin (Li et al., 2022), albeit most trials settle for 25 mg as a standard dose in adults. The issue of microdosing also needs more scientific scrutiny, albeit the evidence for efficacy is generally regarded as low (see below).

For the other psychedelics, evidence is such that we can conclude that a number are 'promising' and mostly appear safe (though ibogaine has particular issues, as outlined in Chapter 7). Thus, much more work is required, and each new molecule that is discovered or developed needs to be subjected to rigorous testing. Furthermore, questions remain as to how products extracted from plants can be tested as discrete molecules, as arguably some of the effects are due to complex interactions of diverse chemicals within the plant, as has been seen for cannabis. Ayahuasca is particularly challenging in this regard, being a mixture of two plants, usually brewed into a tea.

Issues of efficacy in other disorders

The range of psychiatric disorders for which PAP has been investigated is impressive in terms of breadth, but there are many other disorders that deserve attention. Review of registered trials (Figure 11.2) shows the extent of interest across mental health and addictions, in terms of treatment targets. This raises interesting considerations regarding which agent(s) have efficacy for which disorder(s) and the extent of cross-disorder efficacy. For example, whilst most PAP trials using MDMA have been in people with PTSD, there have been robust benefits for mood symptoms as well. Thus, PAP has the potential to target more than one symptom set at a time, albeit that is hardly unique in terms of therapies for mental health problems (e.g. most antidepressant also have benefit for anxiety symptoms, and a number of atypical antipsychotics can have antidepressant effects).

What is perhaps more innovative is that there is also scope for treating comorbid disorders simultaneously, with PAP. For example, a proposed trial of DMT will enrol people with comorbid major depression, alcohol use disorder, and dual diagnosis (see Chapter 6). This is a relatively novel approach in that most trials of mental disorders exclude people with substance use disorders, and vice versa, despite such comorbidities being extremely common in clinical practice. A further example is the potential for MDMA to address eating disorders in people with PTSD (Brewerton et al., 2021). Thus, there is an opportunity for PAP trials to address important questions regarding comorbid conditions, and thus inform clinically relevant treatment approaches. It does raise a raft of methodological questions, though, including which component of the intervention is actually effective for which symptoms or behaviours, how changes in one symptom set impact other symptoms and behaviours, how to define primary vs. secondary outcomes, and how to estimate effect sizes for different outcomes and determine sample sizes for adequate power for potentially differential outcomes.

Safety issues

As discussed in Chapter 10, although relatively benign in terms of side effects, long-term efficacy and safety of the psychedelics and psychedelic-like agents remain to be established, albeit some reassurance regarding safety can be derived from studies that have investigated long-term users of these agents. For example, as detailed in Chapter 6, surveys of long-term ayahuasca drinkers suggest use over protracted periods is largely well tolerated; the same can be said of psilocybin, and overall the classical psychedelics are ranked low in terms of potential harms to self or society (Bonomo et al., 2019; Nutt et al., 2010). Schlag et al. (2022) have provided a useful recent overview of the field, titled 'Adverse effects of psychedelics: from anecdotes and misinformation to systematic science'.

Ketamine has raised some particular safety issues, including the immediate dissociative effects, tolerance development and abuse potential, neuronal injury (shown in nonhuman primates), and progressive cystitis. It has been suggested that these risks and their sequelae can be largely ameliorated by careful dosing in safe clinical settings, and clinical guidelines have been developed (Bayes et al., 2021).

Of course reliance on retrospective self-report is not as robust as long-term prospective studies, and it has been pointed out that safety signals have such a low incidence in most studies that a very large number of participants would be required to fully interrogate this issue (Perkins et al., 2021). Longer-term follow-up (up to 4.5 years) from RCTs have been performed for psilocybin in end-of-life depression and anxiety (Agin-Liebes et al., 2020). However, those studies are relatively small ($n = 15$), and, given the cross-over design, all participants had exposure to the active dose of psilocybin.

It is also not known what the risks of these agents might be in people with bipolar I disorder or schizophrenia spectrum disorders. Intuitively a personal or family history of these disorders would seem to be sensible exclusion criteria for psychedelics and related agents and have been so in most clinical trials (ketamine has been used in people with bipolar II). But bipolar depression is a major area of unmet need, and whether people with bipolar depression who have suffered for protracted periods and have not responded adequately to conventional treatments should automatically be denied a potentially life-saving therapy remains moot. And it is simply not known how far removed a relative with a history of psychotic disorder must be from the patient for treatment to be considered safe. There is also the problem of 'subthreshold' or 'high-risk' individuals who have a psychotic predisposition and who could theoretically be at risk of precipitation of psychosis by psychedelics and related agents. Defining optimal exclusion criteria for psychedelic studies is an important piece of work that remains to be done.

Further long-term RCTs and pharmacovigilance studies will be important, notably as new agents are developed. Country-based or even international registries of people treated with these agents should be considered.

The need to define the effective neurobiological mechanisms

Whilst much of the interest in psychedelics and related compounds as psychiatric medicines has been driven by clinical efficacy, it has also opened up a raft of questions about neurobiology. These are important to address if we are to use this opportunity to understand better the biological underpinnings of psychiatric and addictive disorders, as well as informing the development of other novel compounds. Ketamine is a dissociative anaesthetic acting through antagonism of the N-methyl-D-aspartic acid (NMDA) receptor, implicating glutamatergic mechanisms. But the fact that certain other antagonists at that receptor do not seem to have antidepressant effects, and that some NMDA agonists have antidepressant properties, raises questions about the exact mechanism of action (Schatzberg, 2014). There is also debate about which ketamine enantiomer is most effective, with a recent review of twenty-four trials (n = 1877) suggesting that racemic ketamine is more effective for depression than esketamine: head-to-head trials are required (Bahji et al., 2021). It has also been suggested that the opioid system is involved, with the demonstration that naltrexone attenuates the antidepressant effect, albeit the implications of this finding are debated (Sanacora, 2019).

MDMA has effects on glutamatergic pathways but also raises levels of oxytocin: it has been questioned as to how much each of these (and other) actions are relevant for its clinical efficacy. There is also evidence for some effects being mediated by the serotonin system, with MDMA demonstrating a moderate affinity for 5-HT_2 and adrenergic α_2 receptors (Nichols, 2000). This is further supported by the 5HT-2 receptor antagonist ketanserin blocking some MDMA effects (though notably NOT positive mood effects) (Liechti et al., 2000). These results suggest that the 5-HT_2 receptors may mediate hallucinogenic like effects, such as the intensification of colours, while the euphoric-type effects of MDMA may be mediated by the release of dopamine or serotonin enhancement at other receptors (e.g. 5-HT1A). Indeed, administration of the D_2 antagonist haloperidol attenuates psychological responses, such as positive mood, while maintaining the cardiovascular responses frequently associated with MDMA (Liechti & Vollenweider, 2000).

For the classic psychedelics, the major postulated antidepressant and antianxiety effects are generally seen as being mediated by 5HT-2A agonism: there are downstream second-messenger effects impacting glutamate and dopamine, and effects on gene expression (González-Maeso et al., 2007; Ling et al., 2022). In research on LSD, for example, it has been shown that subjective effects are mediated by 5HT2A activation (Preller et al., 2017). The primacy of the 5HT-2A effect also gains support from experiments that show that pretreatment with the 5HT-2A antagonist ketanserin blocks the psychedelic effect in humans (Vollenweider, 2001). However, whilst it is generally accepted that 5HT-2A agonism is a necessary component of efficacy for the classical psychedelics, it is still uncertain whether it is in itself sufficient. Different psychedelics have different affinities for the 5HT-2A receptor, as well as other serotonin receptors (e.g. 5HT-2C, 5HT-7), and each individual compound demands scrutiny in this regard.

In terms of effects on brain circuitry, much work has been done to understand effects of the classical psychedelics (LSD, psilocybin, and ayahuasca) on the default mode network, demonstrating reductions in activation of medial prefrontal cortex being correlated with subjective effects. A decreased amygdala response to fear has also been observed, persisting for up to a month. Other effects are also time-bound, and studies of short vs. long-term effects of these agents will be important in elucidating neurobiological underpinning of therapeutic effects (as well as potential unwanted effects). A recent investigation of fMRI data from two depression trials showed a 'global increase in brain network integration' (p844) after psilocybin dosing, which was correlated with improvement in depression scores; the effect was not observed with placebo-dosed psilocybin, or with escitalopram (Daws et al., 2022). Further studies of short- vs. long-term effects of these agents will be important in elucidating neurobiological underpinning of therapeutic effects (as well as potential unwanted effects).

Do we need the psychedelic experience?

Several studies have demonstrated improvements in well-being and creativity using microdosing of psychedelics (Kuypers et al., 2019). However, scientifically sound evidence to support these claims is lacking, and it is a tricky area to investigate. Szigeti et al. (2021) used a highly novel 'self-blinding' approach whereby users of psychedelics (n = 191) incorporated a placebo control into their regime: any benefits for psychedelics over placebo were marginal and potentially impacted by some participants unblinding themselves. The authors conclude that 'anecdotal benefits of microdosing can be explained by the placebo effect' (Szigeti et al. (2021). In the context of psychiatric illness, microdosing has not been sufficiently scientifically scrutinized, albeit ongoing trials are investigating the effects of micro- vs. macrodoses using psilocybin (e.g. National Library of Medicine, 2020). The results from such trials will provide insights into the therapeutic effects of microdosing. However, as discussed throughout this book, it appears that a strong psychedelic experience is a vital component in the therapeutic effects. Thus, it is important for us to determine, through validated measures, what part of the psychedelic experience is critical to therapeutic outcomes.

As it stands, the mechanisms through which positive psychological outcomes occur through the psychedelic 'trip', are not well understood. We know that peak psychedelic experiences have been rated among the most personally meaningful experiences of people's lives (Griffiths et al., 2018) and that the experience of challenging emotional breakthroughs correlate with long-term psychological changes (Roseman et al., 2019). Even the word 'psychedelic' itself means 'revealing the psyche or the soul' (Huxley et al., 1999), so it is clear that there are components of the experience that may be particularly beneficial. However, measuring this remains a difficult challenge, especially given the diverse range of compounds considered psychedelic. Several questionnaires have been developed to measure various aspects (see Box 11.1) including mystical experiences, altered consciousness, challenging experiences, emotional breakthroughs, and psychological insights. Notably, these tend to be secondary measures in clinical trials, and it is difficult to compare experiences across psychedelics and between patients. As the field moves forward, it will be important to understand better what components of a psychedelic experience are crucial to treatment for each psychedelic.

Box 11.1 Examples of measures developed to measure the psychedelic experience

- 5-Dimensional Altered States of Consciousness Questionnaire (5DASC): (Dittrich et al., 2010; Studerus et al., 2010): The newest version of the Altered States of Consciousness questionnaire which was developed in 1998 (Dittrich, 1998). A ninety-four-item, self-report questionnaire using a visual analogue scale ranging from 'No, not more than usually' to 'Yes, much more than usually'. It assesses psychedelic experience in areas such as oceanic boundlessness, anxious ego dissolution, and auditory alterations, among others.
- Challenging Experiences Questionnaire (Barrett et al., 2016): A twenty-six-item, self-report questionnaire using a Likert scale ranging from zero ('None or not at all') to five ('Extreme: more than ever before in my life'). Assesses challenging experiences in seven domains: grief, fear, death, insanity, isolation, physical distress, and paranoia.
- Emotional Breakthrough Inventory (Roseman et al., 2019): A six-item, self-report questionnaire assessing resolving personal conflict and emotional release on a visual analogue scale ranging from zero ('No, not more than usual') to one hundred ('Yes, entirely or completely'). It is a dose-dependent questionnaire that can potentially help predict positive psychological outcomes after a psychedelic experience.
- Mystical Experiences Questionnaire (Maclean et al., 2012): A thirty-item, self-report questionnaire using a Likert scale ranging from zero ('None') to five ('Extreme'). Assesses psychedelic experience in several domains, including transcendence, positive mood, ineffability, and mystical experiences.
- Psychological Insight Scale (Peill et al., 2022): A six-item questionnaire using a visual analogue scale that assesses personal psychological insight that can emerge after a psychedelic experience.

Understanding what role, if any, nonordinary experiences and subjective experiences play in the healing process can help inform therapists in developing a therapeutic plan that both encourages these experiences and properly prepares patients for when they encounter them.

What should the psychotherapy entail?

The psychotherapeutic component of PAP is addressed in Chapter 2. Suffice to say, the protocols vary across studies, but mostly include a number of preparatory sessions, one or more dosing sessions, and a series of integrative sessions. The preparatory sessions seem to be important in establishing a trusting therapeutic alliance and reducing the likelihood of a 'bad trip' in the dosing sessions. Some studies have used a highly developed manual with intensive training (e.g. MAPS in the PTSD trials), whilst others have employed a less-structured approach (e.g. the Imperial College London study of TRD). Inevitably the processes need some modification across disorders and across substances, and how much of a 'core curriculum' can be devised is not yet determined.

The content and delivery of the psychotherapy has not been empirically compared across studies. As new psychedelic and psychedelic-like substances are investigated, with different types and duration of 'trip' and different side effects associated, the psychotherapy may require adjustment. Also, content of integrative sessions in particular will need to be responsive to different clinical states: for example, in trials of people with obsessive compulsive disorder, it would intuitively seem important to address exposure and response prevention as part of this phase, but again, that requires empirical investigation.

Another unresolved issue is what other components are required for the psychedelic experience to be effective? One consideration is the musical accompaniment, which is generally seen as a key part of the dosing experience, but which can take different forms. Interestingly, Kaelen et al. (2018) in a qualitative study of nineteen participants in a psilocybin TRD study, reported that 'the nature of the music experience was significantly predictive of reductions in depression 1 week after psilocybin, whilst general drug intensity was not' (p505). Investigation of optimal musical experiences that enhance the outcomes of PAP should be a focus of future research.

What is the ideal trial design?

Apart from obvious issues germane to all clinical trials, including randomized controlled experimental designs that are sufficiently powered to detect meaningful and realistic effect sizes, there are a number of special considerations in PAP trials. One major factor is representativeness. For example, the TRD trial of Carhart-Harris et al. (2016) enrolled mostly people who self-referred after seeing media about the study, introducing inevitable expectancy bias. Given the high level of public interest in the topic, and other factors alluded to above, this will remain an issue for future studies, and some measure of it is warranted. There is also the problem of what to do at the end of any trial. For responders, how long are effects likely to persist, and what should be done if people relapse? Will redosing be required, and if so, at whose expense? And what of people who fail to respond? They might be at particular risk of suicide, given they have already shown 'resistance' to conventional treatments, and may have an investment in PAP being the 'answer'. Thus, aftercare is an important consideration.

But perhaps the most difficult parameter to deal with in terms of RCTs of PAP lies in how blinding of patient and practitioner can be maintained. Participants in PAP trials generally guess accurately as to whether they are receiving active compound or placebo. Mithoefer et al. (2018) looked at this across varying doses of MDMA in PTSD and found participants could recognize active compound with

> **Box 11.2** Potential comparator agents for use in trials of psychedelics and psychedelic-like compounds
>
> - Inert placebo: issues of blinding
> - Low dose of the active compound: this has been used with MDMA (see above) as well as psilocybin
> - Methamphetamine: this has marked prosocial effects and can cause dangerous reactions, including psychosis
> - Methylphenidate: a stimulant
> - Modafinil: also a stimulant with potential physiological and psychologic adverse effects
> - Niacin: causes a skin flush but no particular psychological effects
> - Benzodiazepines: anxiolytic, and a very different psychological effect compared with the psychedelic experience—used in several ketamine trials
> - Diphenhydramine: an antihistamine with sedative effects

85% accuracy at a dose of 100 mg and 77% at 40mg. Thus, low dose was still not effective at blinding, and actually exacerbated participants' anxiety levels and led to poorer outcomes. Various options for an appropriate control agent are shown in Box 11.2.

Thus, there is no perfect way of blinding participants in PAP trials. Inert placebo or a very low dose of the active agent (e.g. 1 mg psilocybin) seem most pragmatic. Asking people as to whether they have been able to recognize whether they have received the active dose is useful, but the timing of such questions needs to be carefully thought through.

Ethical issues

As noted throughout this book, psychedelic experiences, especially those associated with psilocybin, LSD, 5-MeO-DMT, and ayahuasca, can manifest as a wide-range of effects on human consciousness and perception. While there are commonalities amongst these experiences, it can be difficult to convey to patients exactly what to expect both during and after taking a psychedelic. For example, explaining the possibility of transcending reality during PAP or discussing the potential for identity transformation after a psychedelic experience can be difficult for patients to understand, especially those who are psychedelic-naïve or mentally ill. This leaves us with an interesting question about the consent process: how can we ensure patients have an informed understanding of their potential experiences and outcomes prior to 'signing up' to PAP? Some commentators have suggested that an expanded consent process that goes above and beyond typical consent may be necessary (Smith & Sisti, 2021). This expanded type of consent may involve videos of the administration session or involving previous patients in the consent process. It has also been suggested that the preparatory therapy session, where patients learn about the range of possible experiences, be viewed as extension of the informed-consent process (Smith & Sisti, 2021).

The problem of informed consent is further complicated when we consider the enthusiasm that patients and practitioners may have regarding psychedelics. Patients expecting a 'life-changing' experience based on information portrayed through the media may have unrealistic expectations prior to starting PAP that could leave them disappointed and more vulnerable after treatment. On the other hand, enthusiastic researchers and therapists who are highly engaged may unintentionally set these expectations.

As outlined above, there is also the issue of placebos. Receiving a placebo during a clinical trial may result in significant frustration and even anger, especially for patients who already have a preconceived notion that the intervention could be 'life-changing'. Therapists also may not be as engaged in a session where it is clear that a patient has been given a placebo. In both cases the nocebo effect can emerge so magnifying the active-placebo difference. Therefore, researchers and therapists need to be cognizant of how the media and their biases contribute to the overestimation of potential benefits and the repercussions that this can have on patient health and trial outcomes.

Additionally, there are unique boundary issues that need to be considered in the context of psychedelics. We know psychedelics have the potential to disrupt one's thought process, making it difficult for patients to understand information and make informed decisions while under the influence. This is further impacted by the high level of vulnerability and suggestibility of patients during and after PAP. Addressing in advance a patient's boundaries (e.g. Does the patient want their hand to be held if they are feeling distressed?) before PAP will help in ensuring patients can make informed decisions about their care, and in creating an atmosphere of trust during the experience. On a larger scale, the psychedelic research community should develop a harmonized protocol for therapeutic touch that provides guidance to therapists that encounter these situations. Monitoring patient-therapist interactions during the trip is important to prevent any suggestions of inappropriate touch that might emerge afterwards. Group therapy would also minimize this risk but carries other logistic and privacy problems.

Finally, as outlined above, although psychedelics appear to be safe from a psychological and physiological standpoint when administered in clinical settings, RCTs to date have largely excluded individuals considered to be at high risk for adverse effects (schizophrenia, personality disorders, bipolar disorder) in addition to those who have certain comorbidities such as addiction problems. This begs questions not only about how far published research findings can be generalized, but also who should be excluded from PAP? And more importantly, how can we develop research protocols that are more inclusive and representative of the general population while maintaining the safety of patients? These questions among others will need to be answered as the field of psychedelics continues to expand. An important point is that psychedelics such as psilocybin and MDMA are not addictive, though ketamine can be. This suggests serotonin may be protective against addiction, and indeed psilocybin has been shown effective in treating both tobacco and alcohol dependence (see Chapter 3).

How do we bring these agents into mainstream practice?

It is fair to say that there are numerous challenges as to how PAP can be brought into clinical practice. Arguably current trial designs (preparatory sessions, dosing sessions (up to eight hours each) and integration sessions) with two 'therapists' (one of each sex) will prove prohibitive, cost- and timewise, for most centres. Different jurisdictions across the globe will have different healthcare systems, but it is probably true that none has a model that lends itself readily to the clinical or fiscal realities of delivering PAP. Much can be learnt (for good and ill) from the experience with ketamine clinics, which have mushroomed and have sometimes been associated with suboptimal practices. There are also cost considerations for the patient, particularly for those who are financially constrained. A course of MDMA-assisted psychotherapy has been estimated to cost more than US$7,000 per patient, and those with other substances may be much more expensive (Marseille et al., 2020). Though given the huge economic burden of treatment-resistant mental health and addiction problems, this may still be good value for money. However, the cost burden on institutions and on patients need to be reflected in future decisions as we move into the next stages of the psychedelic movement.

Questions about therapeutic training also need to be addressed before these agents are brought into mainstream practice. It will be important to parse out what is critical in PAP and how these components can be organized into training for therapists. Will therapists be trained to administer PAP for all psychedelics, and will specific training courses be required for each medication and each target disorder? More importantly, will training courses be mandated, and what, if any, prerequisites should be required to take them? Training will also need to be considered in the context of costs to ensure that if a training program is put in place, it is not cost-prohibitive for either the institution or the therapists. Currently, there are some institutions such as the California Institute of Integral Studies and MAPS that have established training programs and certificates for psychedelic therapies. It is safe to assume that more of these programs will be developed in the future, and issues of quality of content, eligibility, and credentialing will need to be carefully considered. The recent decision by the State of Oregon to legalize magic mushrooms and make therapy with them available across the state by 2023 raises a new and very interesting model of publicly funded psychedelic therapy.

Finally, there also needs to be consideration taken of how psychedelics will appear in mainstream practice. Will advertising be allowed? What will the safety parameters be for storage and dispensing? Will there be stipulations about the medical workup and availability of medical support during dosing, if required? And will the agents be required to always be used with the psychotherapeutic 'wrap-around'? These issues will need to be informed by input from all stakeholders, including patients and carers.

REFERENCES

Agin-Liebes GI, Malone T, Yalch MM, et al. (2020) Long-term follow-up of psilocybin-assisted psychotherapy for psychiatric and existential distress in patients with life-threatening cancer. Journal of Psychopharmacology 34:155–166.

Bahji A, Vazquez GH, Zarate CA Jr (2021) Comparative efficacy of racemic ketamine and esketamine for depression: a systematic review and meta-analysis. Journal of Affective Disorders 278:542–555.

Barrett FS, Bradstreet MP, Leoutsakos JS, et al. (2016) The Challenging Experience Questionnaire: characterization of challenging experiences with psilocybin mushrooms. Journal of Psychopharmacology 30:1279–1295.

Bayes A, Dong V, Martin D, et al. (2021) Ketamine treatment for depression: a model of care. Australian and New Zealand Journal of Psychiatry 55:1134–1143.

Bogenschutz MP, Ross S, Bhatt S, et al. (2022) Percentage of heavy drinking days following psilocybin-assisted psychotherapy vs placebo in the treatment of adult patients with alcohol use disorder: a randomized clinical trial. JAMA Psychiatry 79(10):953–962. doi:10.1001/jamapsychiatry.2022.2096.

Bonomo Y, Norman A, Biondo S, et al. (2019) The Australian drug harms ranking study. Journal of Psychopharmacology 33:759–768.

Brewerton TD, Lafrance A, Mithoefer MC (2021) The potential use of N-methyl-3,4-methylenedioxyamphetamine (MDMA) assisted psychotherapy in the treatment of eating disorders comorbid with PTSD. Medical Hypotheses 146:110367.

Carhart-Harris R, Giribaldi B, Watts R, et al. (2021) Trial of psilocybin versus escitalopram for depression. New England Journal of Medicine 384:1402–1411.

Carhart-Harris RL, Bolstridge M, Rucker J, et al. (2016) Psilocybin with psychological support for treatment-resistant depression: an open-label feasibility study. Lancet Psychiatry 3:619–627.

Davis AK, Barrett FS, May DG, et al. (2021) Effects of psilocybin-assisted therapy on major depressive disorder: a randomized clinical trial. JAMA Psychiatry 78:481–489.

Daws R, Timmermann C, Giribaldi B, et al. (2022) Increased global integration in the brain after psilocybin therapy for depression. Nature Medicine 28:844–851.

Dittrich A (1998) The standardized psychometric assessment of altered states of consciousness (ASCs) in humans. Pharmacopsychiatry 31(Suppl 2):80–84.

Dittrich A, Lamparter D, Maurer M (2010) 5D-ASC: questionnaire for the assessment of altered states of consciousness. A short introduction. PSIN PLUS.

Goldberg SB, Pace BT, Nicholas CR, et al. (2020) The experimental effects of psilocybin on symptoms of anxiety and depression: a meta-analysis. Psychiatry Research 284:112749.

González-Maeso J, Weisstaub NV, Zhou M, et al. (2007) Hallucinogens recruit specific cortical 5-HT2A receptor-mediated signaling pathways to affect behavior. Neuron 53:439–452.

Goodwin GM, Aaronson ST, Alvarez O, et al. (2022) Single-dose psilocybin for a treatment-resistant episode of major depression. New England Journal of Medicine 387:1637–1648.

Griffiths RR, Johnson MW, Richards WA, et al. (2018). Psilocybin-occasioned mystical-type experience in combination with meditation and other spiritual practices produces enduring positive changes in psychological functioning and in trait measures of prosocial attitudes and behaviors. Journal of Psychopharmacology 32:49–69.

Huxley A, Horowitz M, Palmer C (1999) Moksha: Aldous Huxley's classic writings on psychedelics and the visionary experience. Inner Traditions/Bear.

Kaelen M, Giribaldi B, Raine J, et al. (2018) The hidden therapist: evidence for a central role of music in psychedelic therapy. Psychopharmacology (Berlin) 235:505–519.

Kaur U, Pathak BK, Singh A, Chakrabarti SS (2021) Esketamine: a glimmer of hope in treatment-resistant depression. European Archives of Psychiatry and Clinical Neurosciences 271:417–429.

Kuypers KP, Ng L, Erritzoe D, et al. (2019) Microdosing psychedelics: more questions than answers? An overview and suggestions for future research. Journal of Psychopharmacology 33:1039–1057.

Li NX, Hu YR, Chen WN, Zhang B (2022) Dose effect of psilocybin on primary and secondary depression: a preliminary systematic review and meta-analysis. Journal of Affective Disorders 296:26–34.

Liechti ME, Saur MR, Gamma A, Hell D, Vollenweider FX (2000) Psychological and physiological effects of MDMA ('ecstasy') after pretreatment with the 5-HT2 antagonist ketanserin in healthy humans. Neuropsychopharmacology 23:396–404.

Liechti ME, Vollenweider FX (2000) Acute psychological and physiological effects of MDMA ('ecstasy') after haloperidol pretreatment in healthy humans. European Neuropsychopharmacology 10:289–295.

Ling S, Ceban F, Lui LMW, et al. (2022) Molecular mechanisms of psilocybin and implications for the treatment of depression. CNS Drugs 36:17–30.

Maclean KA, Leoutsakos J-MS, Johnson MW, Griffiths RR (2012) Factor analysis of the Mystical Experience Questionnaire: a study of experiences occasioned by the hallucinogen psilocybin. Journal for the Scientific Study of Religion 51:721–737.

Marseille E, Kahn JG, Yazar-Klosinski B, Doblin R (2020) The cost-effectiveness of MDMA-assisted psychotherapy for the treatment of chronic, treatment-resistant PTSD. PLoS One 15:e0239997.

Mitchell JM, Bogenschutz M, Lilienstein A, et al. (2021) MDMA-assisted therapy for severe PTSD: a randomized, double-blind, placebo-controlled phase 3 study. Nature Medicine 27:1025–1033.

Mithoefer MC, Mithoefer AT, Feduccia AA, et al. (2018) 3,4-methylenedioxymethamphetamine (MDMA)-assisted psychotherapy for post-traumatic stress disorder in military veterans, firefighters, and police officers: a randomised, double-blind, dose-response, phase 2 clinical trial. Lancet Psychiatry 5:486–497.

National Library of Medicine (US) (2020) The safety and efficacy of psilocybin in participants with treatment resistant depression (P-TRD). Identifier: NCT03775200. https://clinicaltrials.gov/ct2/show/ NCT03775200.

Nichols DE (2000) Role of serotoninergic neurons and 5-HT receptors in the action of hallucinogens, in HG Baumgarten, M Göthert, eds., Serotoninergic neurons and 5-HT receptors in the CNS. Springer, 563–585.

Nutt D (2020) Nutt uncut. Waterside Press.

Nutt DJ, King LA, Phillips LD (2010) Drug harms in the UK: a multicriteria decision analysis. Lancet 376:1558–1565.

Peill JM, Trinci KE, Kettner H, et al. (2022) Validation of the Psychological Insight Scale: a new scale to assess psychological insight following a psychedelic experience. Journal of Psychopharmacology 36:31–45.

Perkins D, Sarris J, Rossell S (2021) Medicinal psychedelics for mental health and addiction: advancing research of an emerging paradigm. Australian and New Zealand Journal of Psychiatry 55:1127–1133.

Phelps J, Shah RN, Lieberman JA (2022) The rapid rise in investment in psychedelics-cart before the horse. JAMA Psychiatry 79(3):189–190. doi:10.1001/jamapsychiatry.2021.3972.

Preller KH, Herdener M, Pokorny T, et al. (2017) The fabric of meaning and subjective effects in LSD-induced states depend on serotonin 2A receptor activation. Current Biology 27:451–457.

Roseman L, Haijen E, Idialu-Ikato K, et al. (2019, Sep). Emotional breakthrough and psychedelics: validation of the Emotional Breakthrough Inventory. Journal of Psychopharmacology 33:1076–1087.

Rosenblat JD, Carvalho AF, Li M, et al. (2019) Oral ketamine for depression: a systematic review. Journal of Clinical Psychiatry 80:13514.

Sanacora G (2019) Caution against overinterpreting opiate receptor stimulation as mediating antidepressant effects of ketamine. American Journal of Psychiatry 176:249.

Schatzberg AF (2014) A word to the wise about ketamine. American Journal of Psychiatry 171:262–264.

Schlag AK, Aday J, Salam I, et al. (2022) Adverse effects of psychedelics: from anecdotes and misinformation to systematic science. Journal of Psychopharmacology 36(3):258–272. doi.org/10.1177/02698811211069100.

Smith WR, Sisti D (2021) Ethics and ego dissolution: the case of psilocybin. Journal of Medical Ethics 47:807–814.

Studerus E, Gamma, A, Vollenweider FX (2010) Psychometric evaluation of the Altered States of Consciousness rating scale (OAV). PLoS One 5:e12412.

Szigeti B, Kartner L, Blemings A (2021) Self-blinding citizen science to explore psychedelic microdosing. eLife 10:1–26.

Vollenweider FX (2001) Brain mechanisms of hallucinogens and entactogens. Dialogues in Clinical Neuroscience 3:265–279.

Index

For the benefit of digital users, indexed terms that span two pages (e.g., 52–53) may, on occasion, appear on only one of those pages.

Tables, figures, and boxes are indicated by t, f, and b following the page number

A

adverse events 29–34, 67, 107, 108t, 113–29
alcohol use disorder 4, 8, 21, 29–35, 31t, 47, 53–54, 55, 66, 67, 134
Alles, Gordon 40
Alzheimer's disease 60
Amanita muscaria (muscimol) 95–97
ancient civilizations 3
antiaddictive agents 55, 66, 77, 88–89, 101
anticonvulsants, interaction with psychedelics 123–24
antidepressants, interaction with psychedelics 121–23
antipsychotics, interaction with psychedelics 123–24
anti-Vietnam war movement 5
anxiety therapy 4, 8, 31t, 47, 53–54, 55, 60, 61t, 66, 67, 134
arketamine 103–4
ataxia 87
ayahuasca 65–74
　adverse events 67
　alcohol use disorder 66, 67
　antiaddictive effects 66
　anxiety therapy 66, 67
　borderline personality disorder therapy 66
　botanical decoction 65
　brain effects 68
　'Changed Worldview and New Orientation to Life' 66–67
　childhood trauma 69
　clinical issues 69–70
　clinical research overview 66–67
　depression therapy 66, 67
　drug use therapy 66, 67
　eating disorders therapy 66
　neurobiology 68, 68b
　Parkinson's disease therapy 66
　personality changes 69
　psychedelic-assisted therapy 70
　psychological effects 66–67
　psychopharmacology 67–68
　psychotherapeutic elements 69
　PTSD therapy 66
　religious practices 65
　tourism 65
　wellbeing benefits 66–67

B

'beginners mind' 19, 21
beta-carboline alkaloids 67–68
bipolar disorder 4, 136
black triangle medicines 124–25
blinding issues 35, 140–41
blissful state 53, 60, 96–97
borderline personality disorder therapy 66
boundary issues 142
brain, effects of psychedelics 26, 27–29, 42, 54, 55–57, 68, 104–5, 137–38, see also neuroplasticity

C

cabergoline 119, 120t
cactus plants 3, 98–99
cardiovascular safety 87, 118–21
cave paintings 3
2C-B 98–100
Challenging Experiences Questionnaire 139b
'Changed Worldview and New Orientation to Life' 66–67
childhood adversity/trauma 17, 69
2CI 98–99
clinical trials 29–37, 31t, 41, 43–47, 60, 61t, 66–67, 82–86, 83t, 88, 106–7, 133–35, 140–41
cognitive function 27, 29, 55, 60, 68
comorbid conditions 135
consent 141–42
Controlled Drug Local Intelligence Networks 125
Controlled Substances Act (CSA) 5
cost issues 37, 143
couples therapy 47
critical period plasticity 68
CYP2D6 122

D

dehydronorketamine 104
Delysid 3–5, 53
dementia therapy 60
depression therapy 4, 8, 31t, 34, 37, 53–54, 55, 60, 61t, 66, 67, 106–7, 110, 133, 134
deregulation of psychedelics 8–9
dihydroergotamine 119, 120t

5-Dimensional Altered States of Consciousness Questionnaire (5DASC) 139b
DMT 2, 67, 116t, 117–18, 120t, 135
dopamine 41, 54, 55–57, 67, 82, 97, 100, 137
drug interactions 121–24
drug use therapy 66, 67, see also ibogaine

E

eating disorders therapy 66
Ehrlichman, John 5
Eleusinian mysteries 3
Emotional Breakthrough Inventory 139b
emotion processing 29, 42–43
ergonovine 119, 120t
esketamine 103–4, 106–7
ethical issues 141–43
existential distress and anxiety 29–34, 31t, 134
expectancy effects 35, 36

F

5-Dimensional Altered States of Consciousness Questionnaire (5DASC) 139b
flashbacks 6, 122–23
functional selectivity 26

G

glutamate receptors 26, 54
Grof, Stanislav 47, 48–49

H

hallucinogen persistence perception disorder 6
headache therapy 31t, 60, 61t
heart valve toxic drugs 119, 120t
Hermle, Leo 6–8
hippie subculture 5
history of psychedelics 1–14, 40–41, 53, 75–78, 95–96, 98
HIV/AIDS patients 31t
Hofmann, Albert 3, 53
holistic approach 17
5-HT (serotonin) 4, 42, 78–80, 100, 114, 115, 116t, 120t, 137, 142–43
5-HT2A receptors 26, 27, 54, 116t, 117–21, 120t, 137
hydroxynorketamine 104

I

ibogaine 75–94
  antiaddictive
    properties 77, 88–89
  ataxia and 87
  clinical trials 82–86, 83t, 88
  historical overview 75–78
  Lambarene 76–77
  morphine modulation 80–81
  neurobiology 78–81
  NMDA receptor antagonist 81
  non-hallucinogenic
    analogue 89
  noribogaine 78–81, 82
  oneiric effects 81–82, 85
  opioid withdrawal 82–86
  psychopharmacology 78–82
  QTc prolongation 87
  religious practices 75–76
  safety issues 86–88
  sleep (disorders) 81–82
imaginal exposure 48b
indigenous cultures 3, 65
Indocybin 3–5
informed consent 141–42

J

Jesus Christ, Amanita muscaria
  and 95–96

K

ketamine 103–12
  adverse events 107, 108t
  anxiety induction 108t
  arketamine 103–4
  blood pressure effects 108t
  brain effects 104–5
  clinical trials 106–7, 133
  dehydronorketamine 104
  depression therapy 106–7,
    110, 133
  dissociation effects 108t
  esketamine 103–4, 106–7
  glutamate release 26
  headache induction 108t
  hydroxynorketamine 104
  nasal spray 103–4, 106–7
  nausea induction 108t
  neurobiology 104–5, 136–37
  norketamine 104
  psychopharmacology 103–4
  safety issues 107, 108t, 136
  Spravato® 106–7
  subanaesthetic doses 106

L

Lambarene 76–77
Leary, Timothy 6
lorcaserin 119
LSD (lysergic acid
  diethylamide) 53–64
  alcohol use disorder 53–54, 55
  antiaddictive effects 55
  anxiety therapy 53–54, 55,
    60, 61t

bipolar disorder patients 4
brain effects 54, 55–57
clinical effects 54–55
clinical trials 60, 61t
cluster headache
  treatment 60, 61t
compassionate use 54
Delysid 3–5, 53
dementia therapy 60
depression therapy 53–54, 55,
  60, 61t
discovery 3–4
dosing strategies 53–54
fears of physiological and
  psychological effects 6
flashbacks 6, 122–23
glutamate receptors 54
historical overview 53
5-HT2A receptors 54, 116t,
  117–18, 120t, 137
microdosing 60
neural correlates 55–57
neurobiology 54, 137
psychedelic-assisted
  psychotherapy 60
psychoactive effects 53
psychosomatic disorders
  therapy 53–54
psychotomimetic
  effects 53–54
Schedule 1 status 54
schizophrenia patients 3–4
studies in healthy
  participants 57–60

M

McKenna, Terence 2–3
MDA 39–40
MDMA 39–51
  alcohol use disorder 21, 47
  brain effects 42
  'breakthrough therapy' 45
  chemical structure 40
  clinical trials 41, 43–47, 133
  couples therapy 47
  emotion processing 42–43
  entactogen and empathogen
    qualities 39–40
  historical background 40–41
  imaginal exposure 48b
  monoamine
    neurotransmitters 41–42
  names for 40
  neurobiology 41–43, 137
  neuropsychological
    effects 42, 44
  neurotoxicity 42
  oxytocin 42
  personality changes 45
  psychedelic-assisted
    therapy 19, 20, 21, 39,
    43–49, 133, 143
  psychological effects 39
  PTSD therapy 41, 43–47,
    133
  Schedule 1 status 41
  side-effects 43
  social anxiety therapy 47

measures of psychedelic
  experiences 139b
5-MeO 100–1
mescaline 3, 98–99
methylergonovine 119, 120t
Metzner, Ralph 100–1
microdosing 8–9, 60, 98, 138
migraine 31t
mindset 18–19, 27
MK-Ultra 6
monoamine
  neurotransmitters 41–
    42, 80t
morphine, ibogaine
  modulation 80–81
Multidisciplinary Association
  for Psychedelic Studies
  (MAPS) 43
muscimol 95–97
music 4, 19–20, 70, 140
mystical experiences 8, 53,
  60, 67, 69
Mystical Experiences
  Questionnaire 139b

N

Naranjo, Claudio 40
Nelson, Ken 101
neurobiology 27–29, 41–43,
  54, 68, 68b, 78–81, 104–
  5, 136–38
neuroplasticity 17, 42, 68, 99
neuropsychological effects 42, 44
neurotoxicity 42
nicotinic receptors 78, 80t
Nixon, Richard 5, 6
NMDA receptors 80t, 81, 103–4,
  105b, 136–37
norfenfluramine 119, 120t
noribogaine 78–81, 82
norketamine 104

O

obsessive-compulsive disorder
  therapy 4, 29–34, 31t
oneiric effects 81–82, 85
opioid dependence see ibogaine
opioid receptors 78–81, 80t, 97
oxytocin 42

P

Parkinson's disease therapy 66
pergolide 119, 120t
personality, post-therapy
  changes 22, 45, 69
Peruvian torch 98
Peyote 98
placebo response 29, 142
postmarketing
  pharmacovigilance 124–25
post-traumatic stress disorder
  (PTSD) therapy 16, 41,
  43–47, 66, 133
psilocin 26, 29, 116t, 117–
  18, 120t
psilocybin 25–38

adverse events 29–34, 113–14
aftercare issues 37
alcohol use disorder 29–35, 31t, 134
ancient civilization use 3
antidepressants, interactions 123
anxiety therapy 31t
appetite loss 2
blinding issues 35
brain effects 26, 27–29
clinical trials 29–37, 31t, 134
cognitive function 29
cost issues 37
depression therapy 31t, 34, 37
emotion processing 29
evolutionary role 2–3
existential distress and anxiety 29–34, 31t, 134
expectancy effects 35, 36
function in mushrooms 2
glutamate receptors 26
HIV/AIDS patients 31t
5-HT2A receptors 26, 27, 116t, 117–18, 120t
Indocybin 3–5
migraine therapy 31t
mindset of user 27
obsessive-compulsive disorder 29–34, 31t
overdose 26
placebo response 29
psychopharmacology 26
psychosis-link 26
regulatory status 36, 37
setting of use 27, 36–37
subjective effects 25, 27
tobacco addiction 29–34, 31t
velada ritual 3
psychedelic-assisted psychotherapy (PAP) 15–24, 139–40
alcohol use disorder 8, 21
anxiety therapy 8
ayahuasca-assisted therapy 70
'beginners mind' 19, 21
boundary issues 142
bringing to mainstream clinical practice 143
'collecting experiences' 19
comorbid conditions 135
consent 141–42
coping style of patients 19
cost issues 143
'default position' 19–20
depression therapy 8
drug-assisted session 20–21
ethical issues 141–43
expectation management 18–19
'inside' position 19–20
integration phase 21–22
key life events 19
LSD-assisted therapy 60
MDMA-assisted therapy 19, 20, 21, 39, 43–49, 133, 143
mindset of patients 18–19
music use 19–20, 140
mystical experience evocation 8
patient-led focus 20–21
personality changes following 22
preparation sessions 17–20
psychoeducation 20
psychological flexibility 21–22, 22b
safety issues 20
settings 19
smoking cessation 8
touch during 19, 142
training of therapists 143
two-therapist dyadic pair model 20
psychological effects 6, 39, 66–67
psychological flexibility 21–22, 22b
Psychological Insight Scale 139b
psychopharmacology 26, 67–68, 78–82, 103–4, 115–18
psychosis
psilocybin link 26
psychotomimetic effect of LSD 53–54
psychosomatic disorders therapy 53–54

Q

QTc prolongation 87

R

religious practices 3, 65, 75–76
Rettig, Octavio 101
Risk Evaluation and Mitigation Strategy (REMS) 124–25
risks see adverse events; safety issues

S

Sabina, Maria 3
safety issues 20, 86–88, 107, 108t, 113–29, 135–36
salvinorin A (Salvia divinorum) 97–98
San Pedro 98
Santa Claus 95–96
Schedule 1 status 6, 54, 125
schizophrenia 3–4, 136
selective serotonin reuptake inhibitors (SSRIs) 15, 121–23
serotonin (5-HT) 4, 42, 78–80, 100, 114, 115, 116t, 120t, 137, 142–43
serotonin syndrome 122
setting of use 19, 27, 36–37
Shulgin, Alexander Sasha 40, 98–99
sleep (disorders) 81–82
smoking cessation 8, 29–34, 31t
social anxiety therapy 47
Spravato® 106–7
'Stoned Ape' theory 2–3
Strassman, Rick 6–8

T

talking therapies 16
terminology 1
thalidomide 124–25
toad venom 101
tobacco addiction 8, 29–34, 31t
touch 19, 142
training of therapists 143

V

valvulopathic drugs 119, 120t
velada ritual 3
Vietnam war 5
Vollenweider, Franz 6–8

W

'war on drugs' 5
Wasson, Gordon 3

Y

Yellow Card scheme 124–25

Z

Zeff, Leo 40, 42